"**GOOD MEDICINE** is a collection of cartoons that will tickle your funny bone."
-Rob Portlock (cartoonist; author, "Off the Church Wall"/ InterVarsity Press)

"For smiles, chuckles and wry humor, you'll enjoy a dose of *GOOD MEDICINE* by Bruce Robinson."
-Dr. Bob Phillips (author, "World's Greatest Collection of Clean Jokes"/ Harvest House)

"Here is a book that exposes the realities of church life in a way that is both humorous and to the point. Anyone who is a pastor, church leader or even a pew warmer will enjoy this book."
-Kelly Gallagher (director/ Beacon Hill Press)

"**Funnier cartoons hath no man made.**" **Stayskal 1:1**
-Wayne Stayskal (editorial cartoonist; creator, *Ralph* [King Features Syndicate])

"Bruce has produced a pile of cartoons aimed to tickle your 'ol funny bone. Here are lots of <u>yucks</u> for your <u>bucks</u>!"

-Doug Jones (cartoonist/illustrator)

"There is some *VERY* clever stuff in here…"
-Ron Wheeler (cartoonist; creator, *The Adventures of Jeremiah*)

"Bruce Robinson's cartoons turn up in journals as diverse as *The Saturday Evening Post* and *National Enquirer*. Enquiring minds will want to know where so many ideas come from. Bruce brings a happily deranged perspective to every subject from angels to ZZZs in a church pew. But why are you reading these lines? The cartoons are much more fun. Have at them!"
-Rob Suggs (editor/cartoonist; author, "It Came From Beneath the Pew"[Intervarsity Press], "The Adventures of Brother Biddle" [Zondervan])

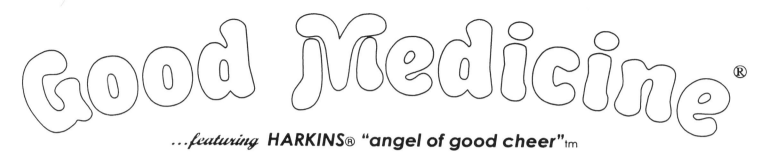

Good Medicine ®

...*featuring* **HARKINS**® *"angel of good cheer"*tm

by

BRUCE ROBINSON

BERCO PRESS
a division of BERCO PUBLISHING
Ft. Lauderdale, Fl.

ISBN: 0-9666956-0-7   Library of Congress Catalog Card Number: 98-96761

Printed in the United States of America   *First Printing: November 1998*

Publisher's Cataloging-in-Publication
(Provided by Quality Books, Inc.)

Robinson, Bruce (Bruce E.), 1956-
    Good Medicine / by Bruce Robinson -- 1st ed.
    p. cm.
    LCCN: 98-96761
    ISBN: 0-9666956-0-7

  1. Christian life--Caricatures and cartoons. 2. Clergy--Caricatures and cartoons. 3. Bible--Caricatures and cartoons. I. Title.

NC1429.R63A4 1998   741.5'973
                           QBI98-1562

In loving memory of William H. & Lois F. Robinson

(and many thanks to my brother Steve for my first drawing table!)

Special thanks to Jim Black and Andrew Persac for your editorial skills.

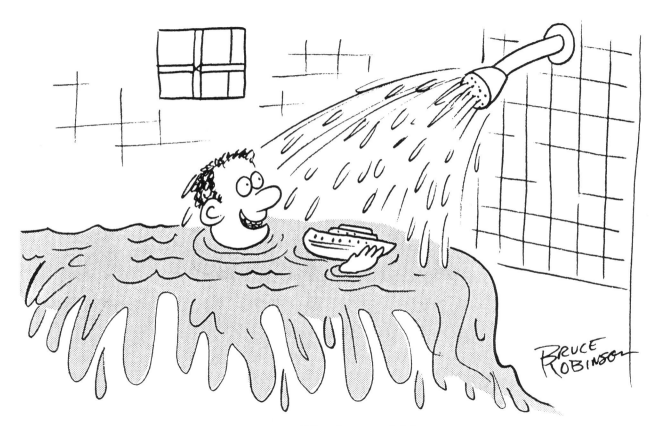

Noah as a kid

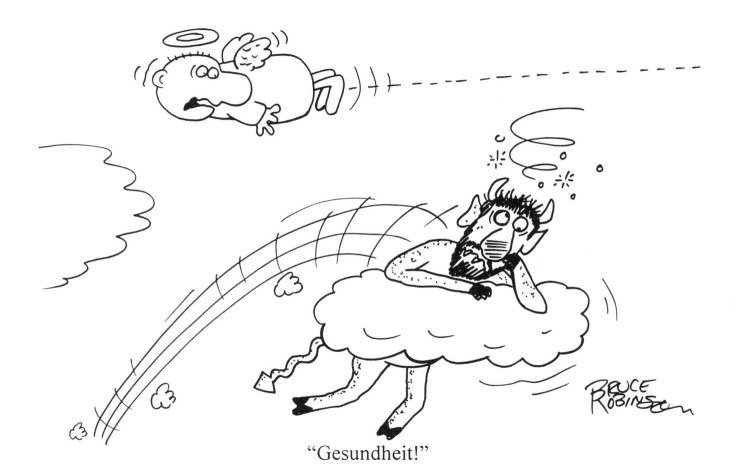

"Gesundheit!"

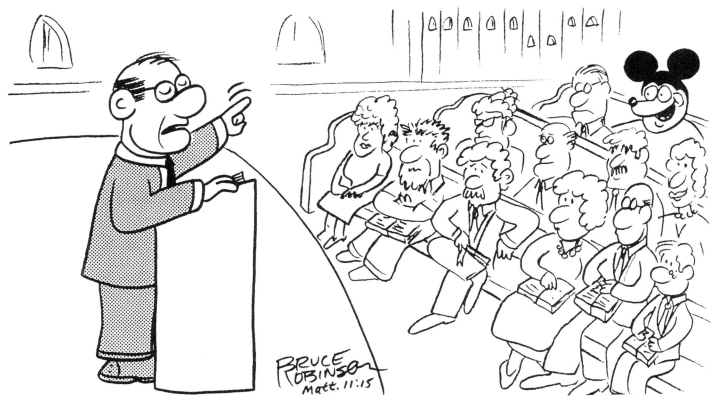

"He who has ears, let him hear..."

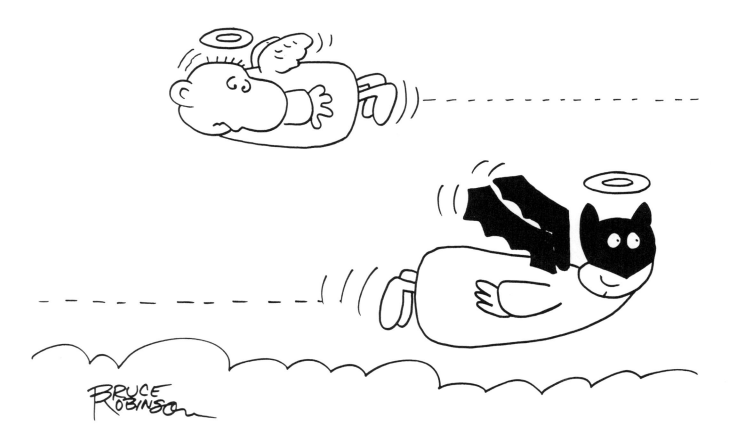

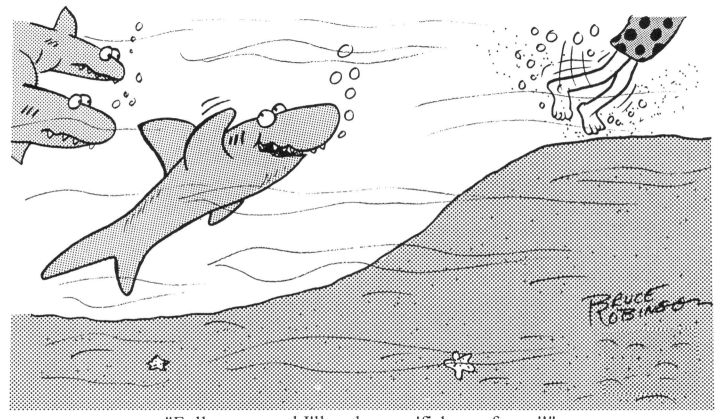

"Follow me and I'll make you 'fishers of men'!"

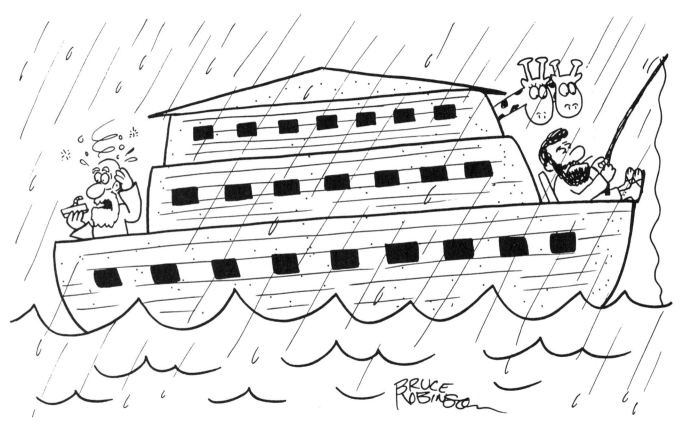

"Hey! Where's the other worm?...I'm missing a worm!"

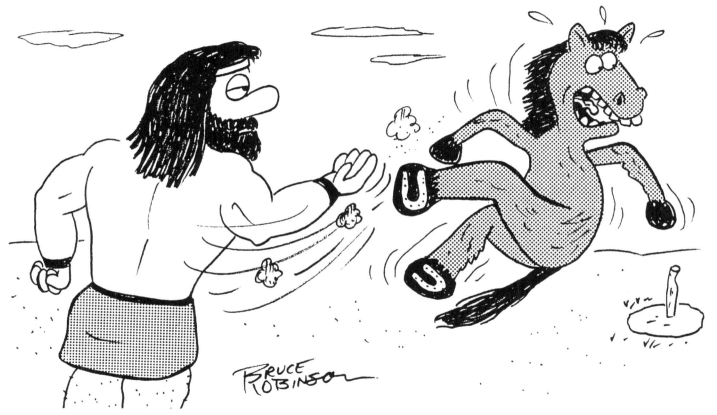

Horseshoes-Samson style

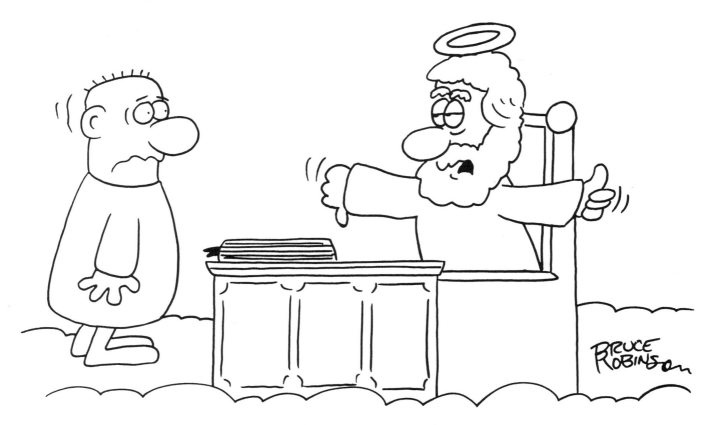

"Smoking or non-smoking?"

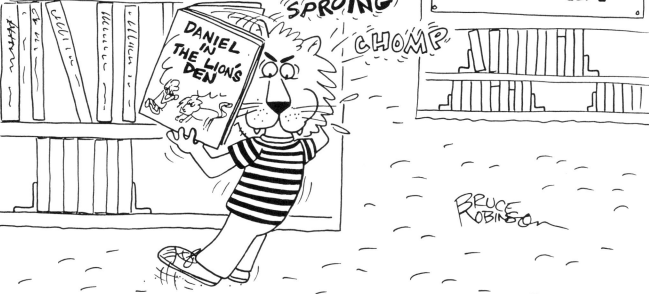

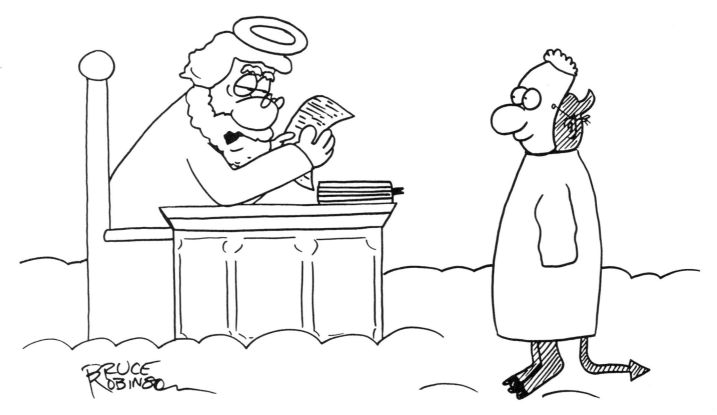

"So you want to see the hot spots, huh?"

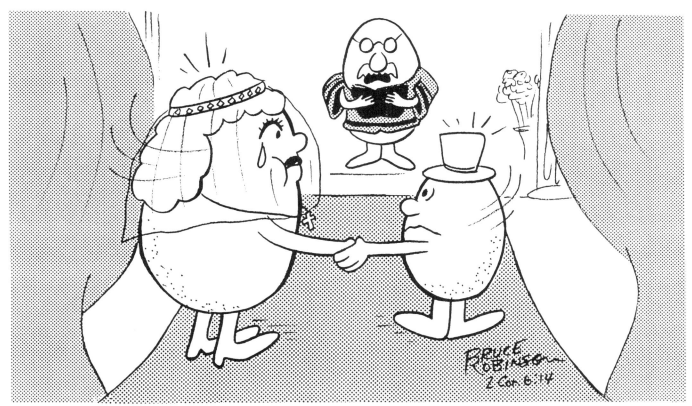

"I'm sorry I can't marry you Humpty-you're unequally yolked."

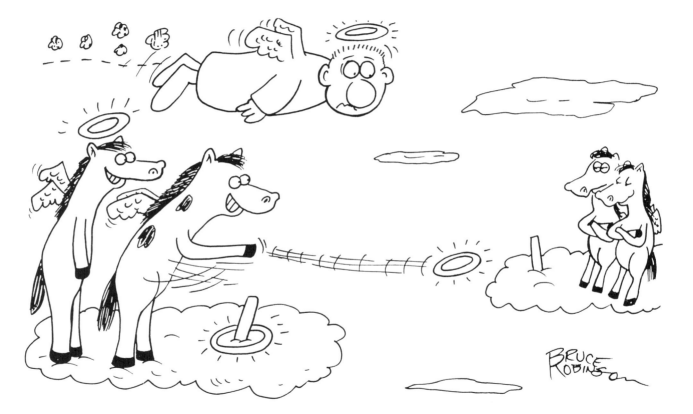

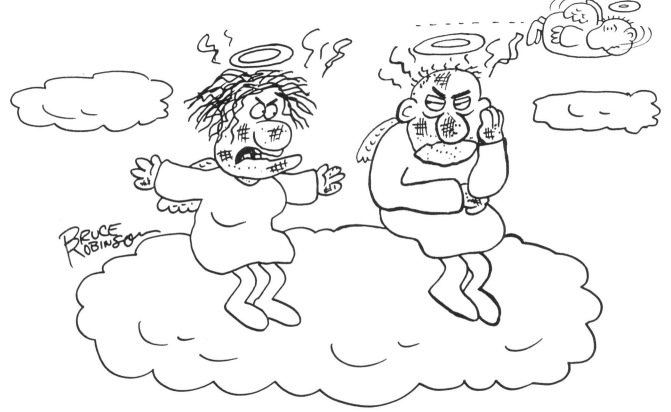

"Quit griping...you said you wanted a light to see why the gas stove wasn't working...well, a match is a light, **isn't** it?!"

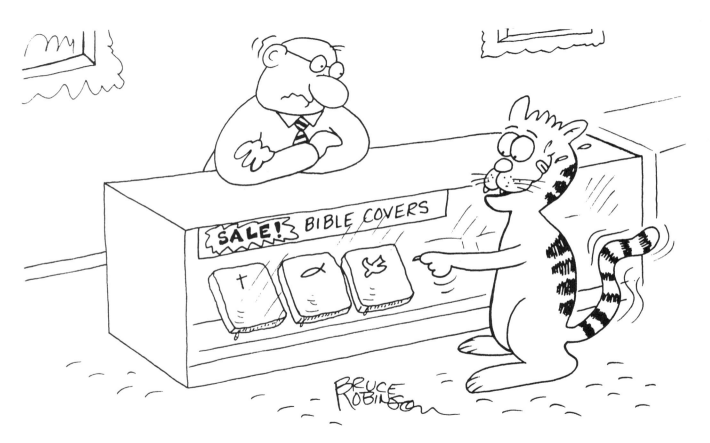

"The cross is nice, but I'm leaning toward the fish or dove."

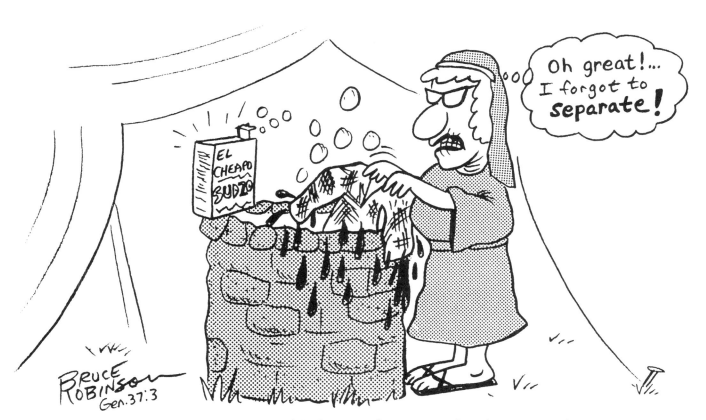

How some say Joseph's 'coat of many colors' came to be

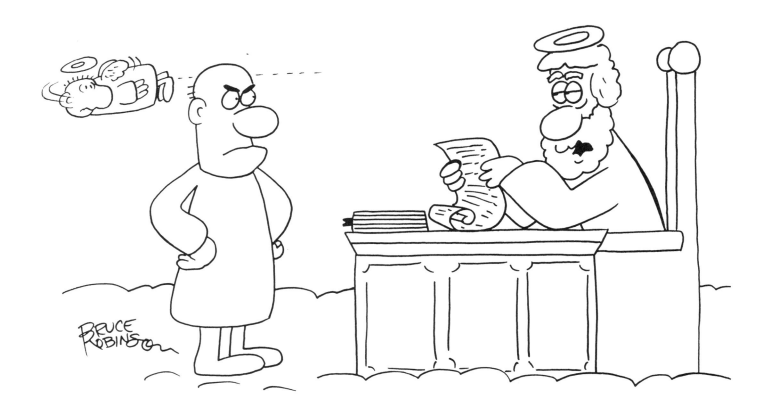

"Now, now Mr. Jones...you can't blame your evil ways on El Niño."

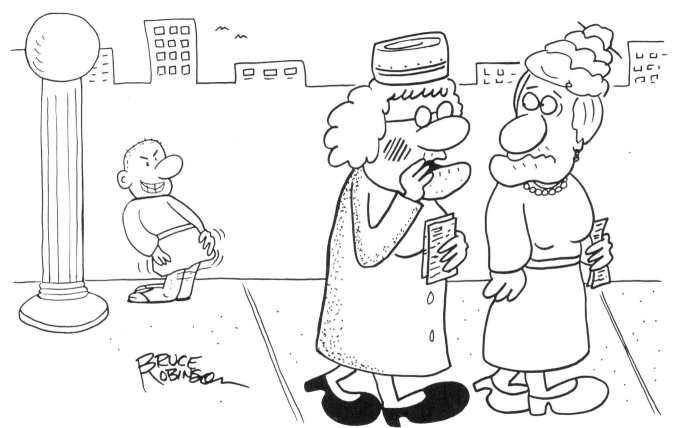

"It's SO embarassing witnessing to 'Moonies'!"

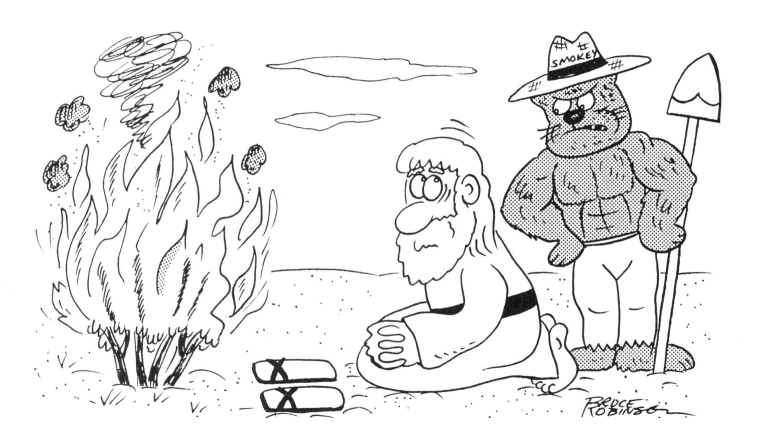

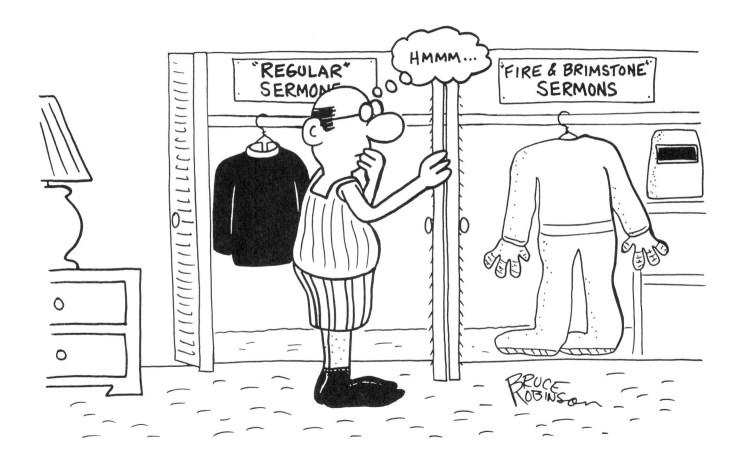

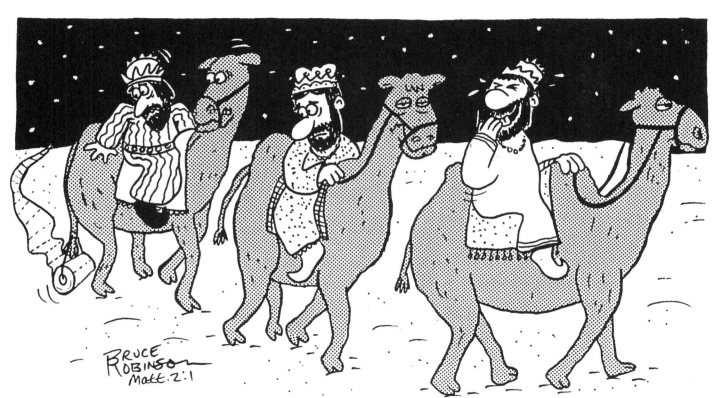

Two wise men & one wise guy

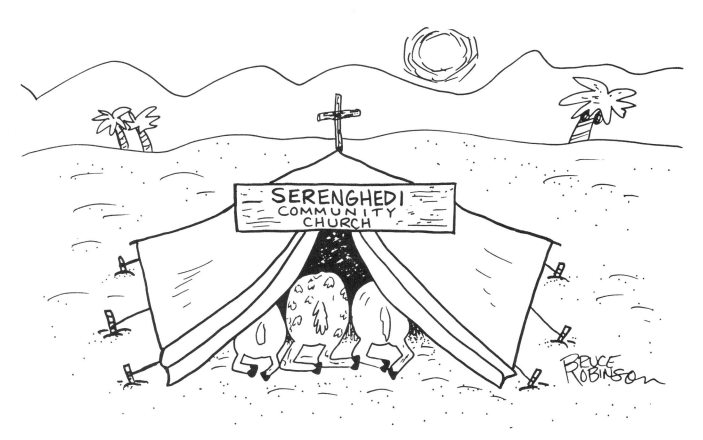

Where the deer and the antelope pray

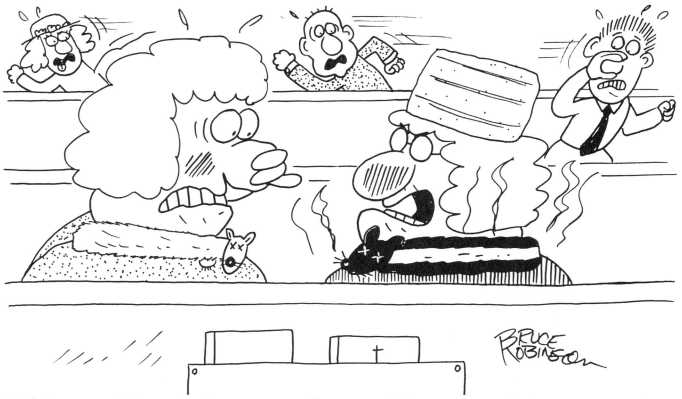

"Life's rotten! Not only has my nose been stuffed-up all week, but some punk at my fur storage place was hassling me just because I wouldn't give him a tip!"

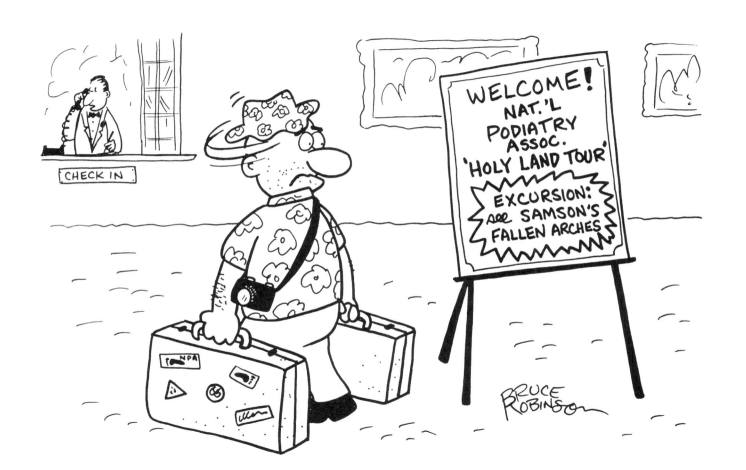

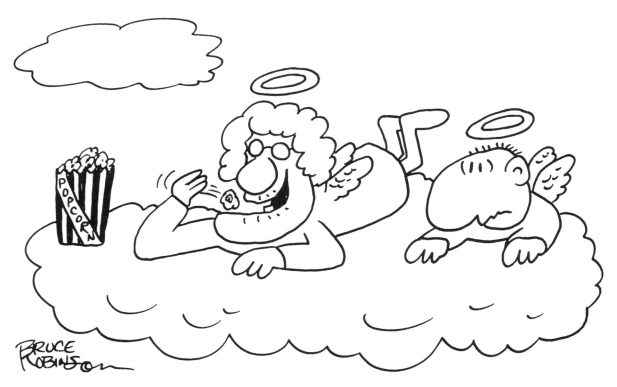

"This oughtta be good...my lawyer's about to read my will...I left everything to my cat, Binky!"

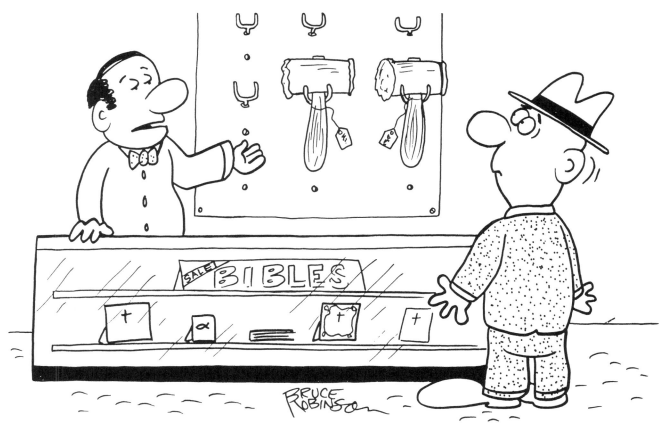

"It's a new witnessing tool for hard-headed prospects."

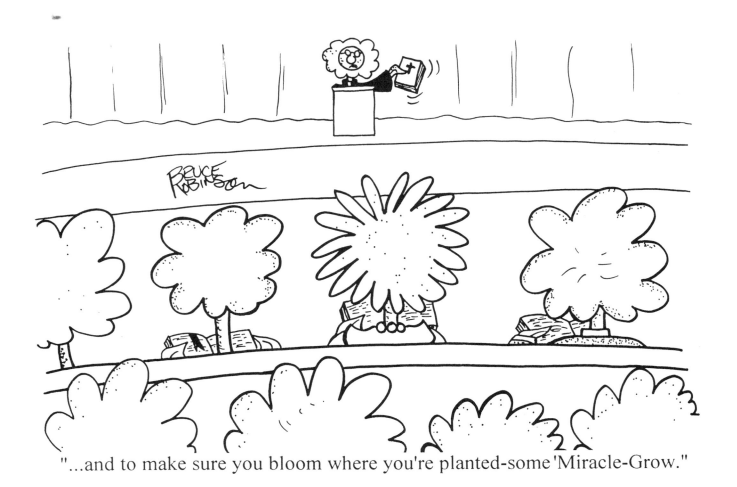

"...and to make sure you bloom where you're planted-some 'Miracle-Grow.'"

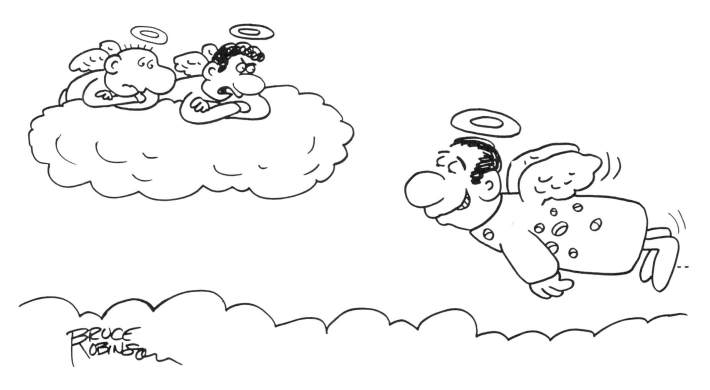

"Oh, here comes Melvin the Martyr. Just because he got here by
a firing squad, he thinks he's 'holier than thou'."

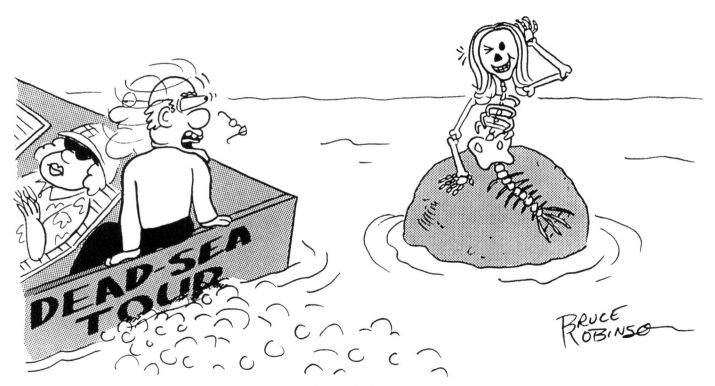

Mermaids of the Dead Sea

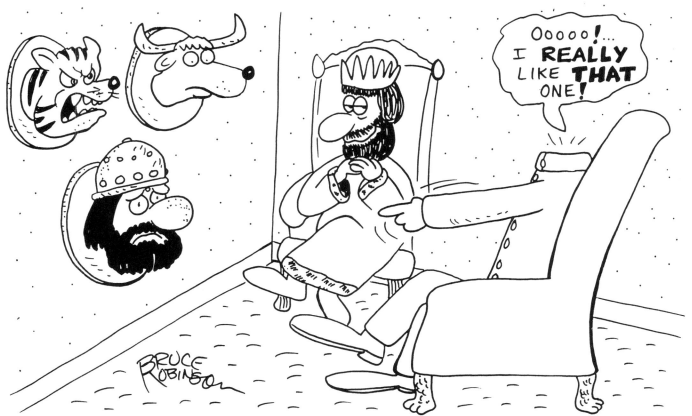

The Headless Horseman visiting King David's trophy room.

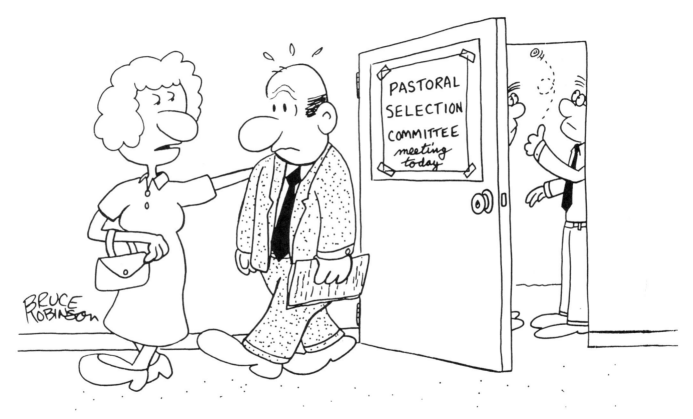

"Don't worry dear- I'm sure they're making their decision with much prayer."

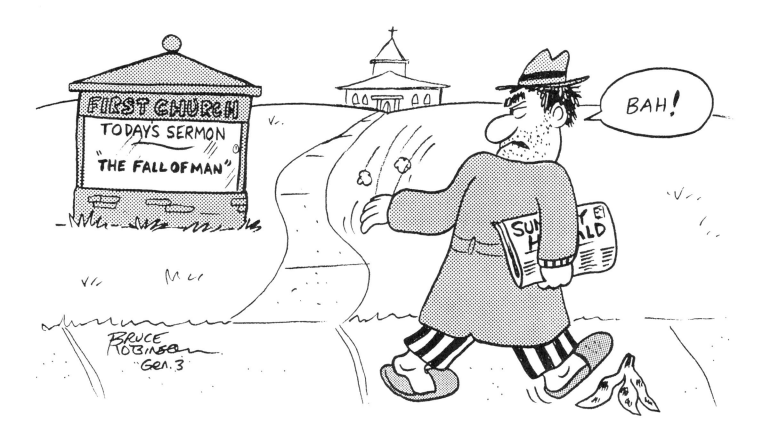

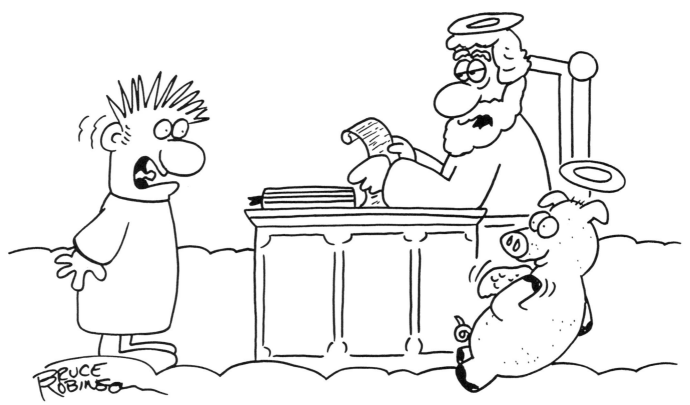

"Since you tithed from the 'net' and not the 'gross', you're going to Hog Heaven instead."

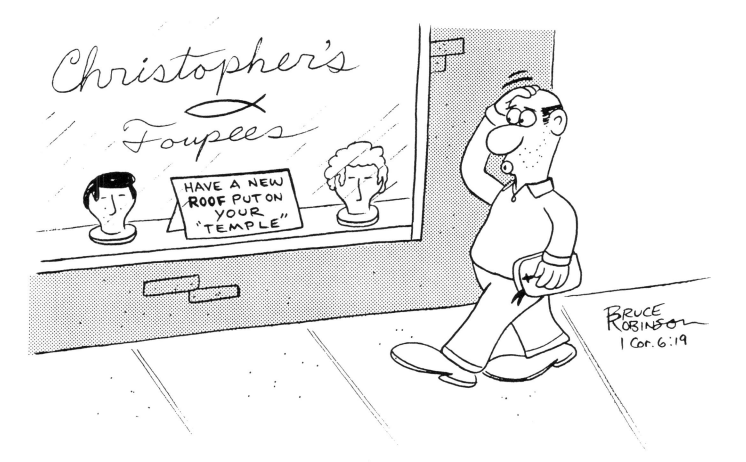

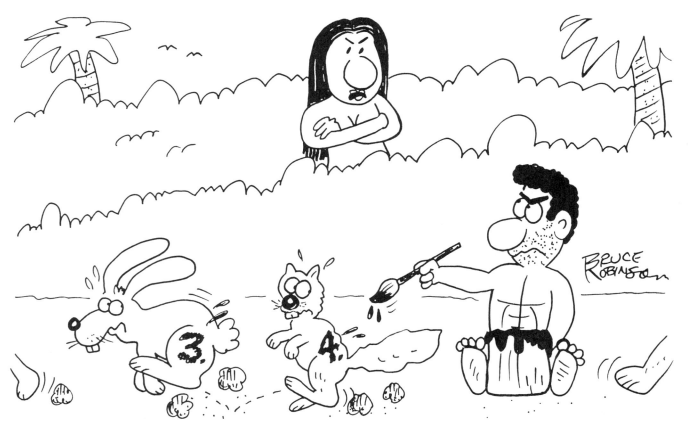

"Adam! Don't be so lazy...God said to NAME them!"

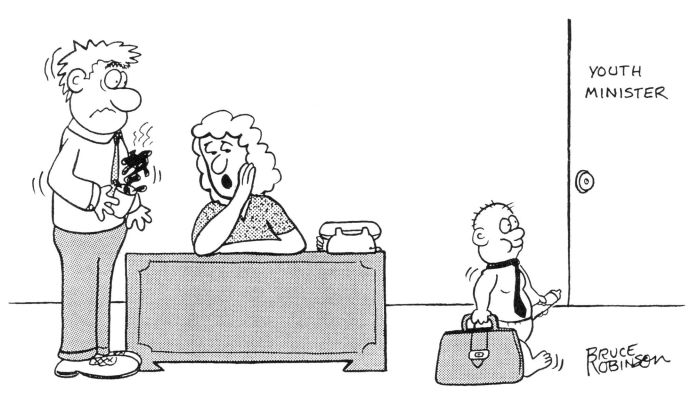

"They say the new youth minister is the youngest one to ever graduate."

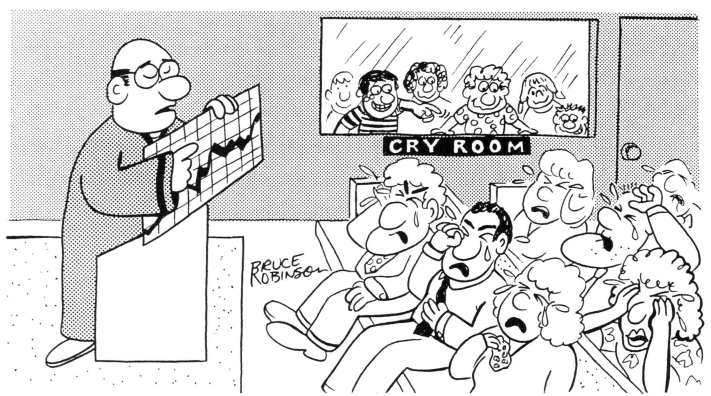

The congregation is told about ANOTHER building fund program

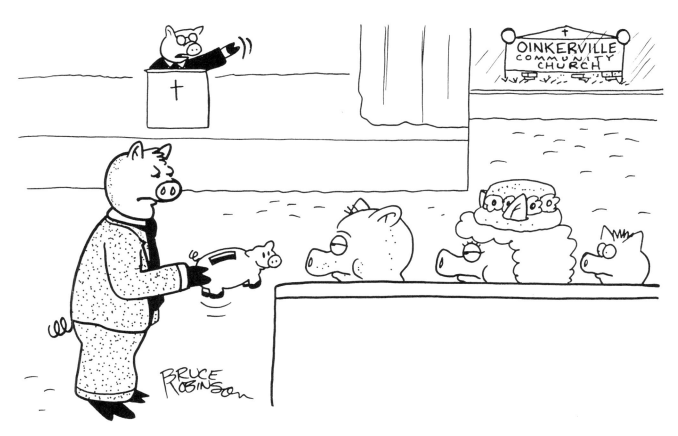

"...and now, the offering."

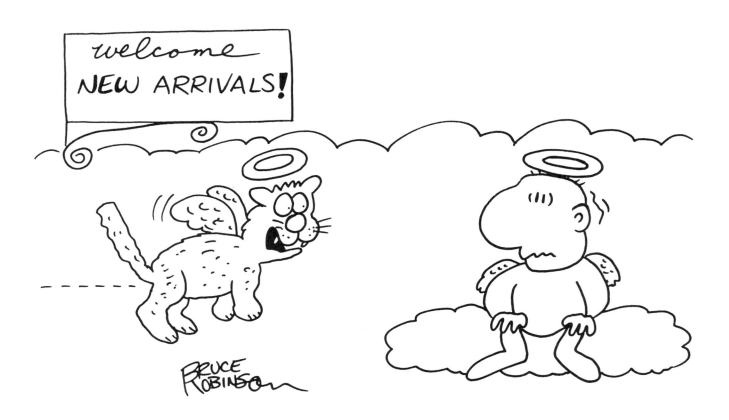

"Someone put quicksand in my litter box."

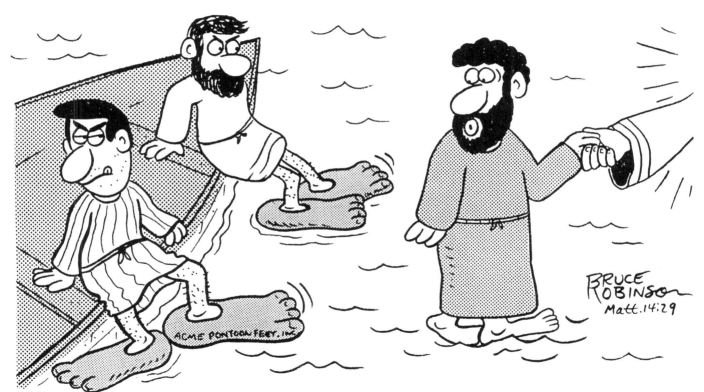

The other disciples were jealous of Peter

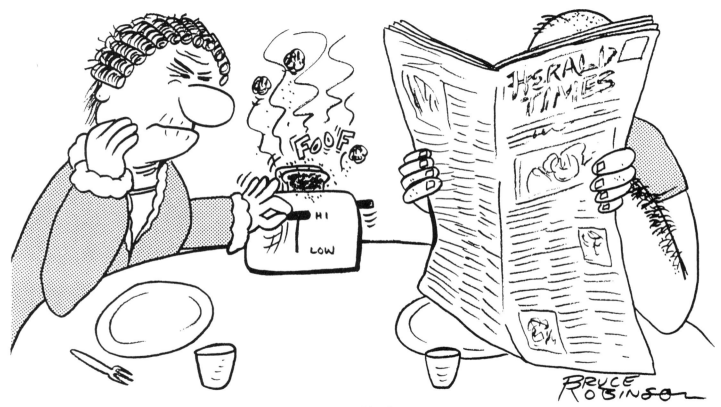

Burnt offerings

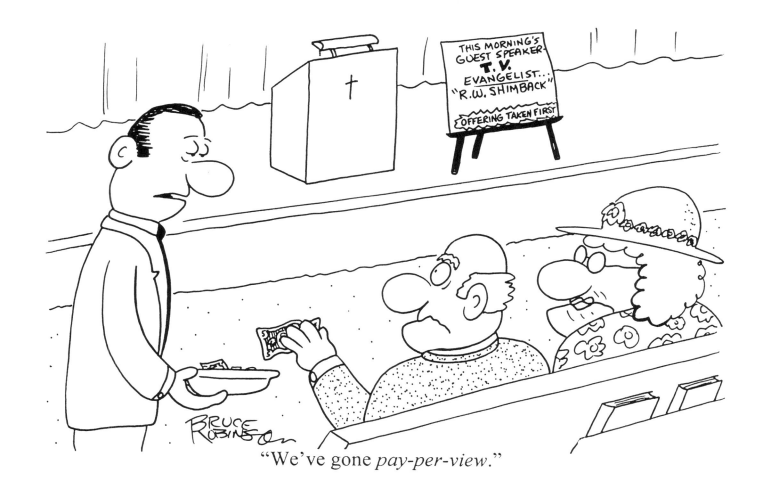

"We've gone *pay-per-view*."

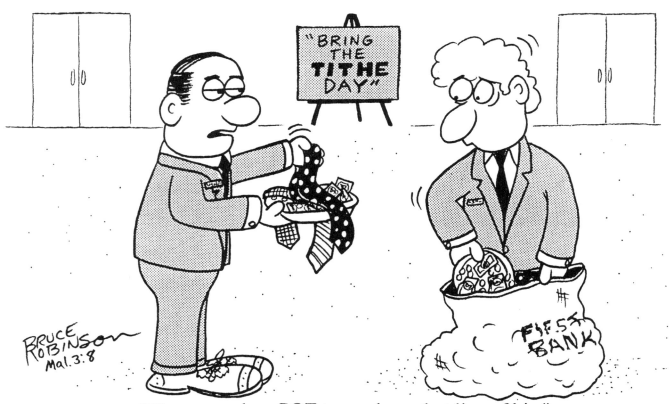

"The pastor has GOT to work on that lisp of his."

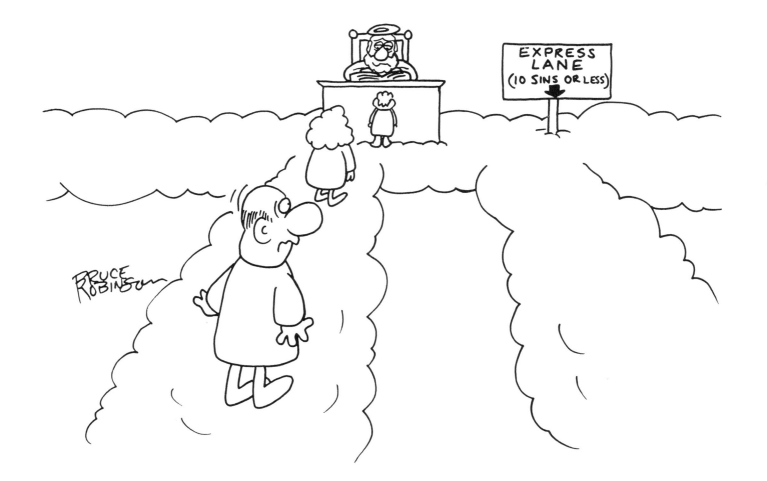

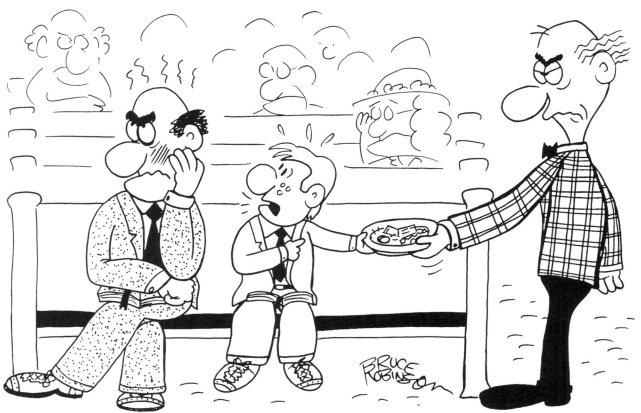

"...but dad!-you said you were gonna give ME that shiny, new quarter!"

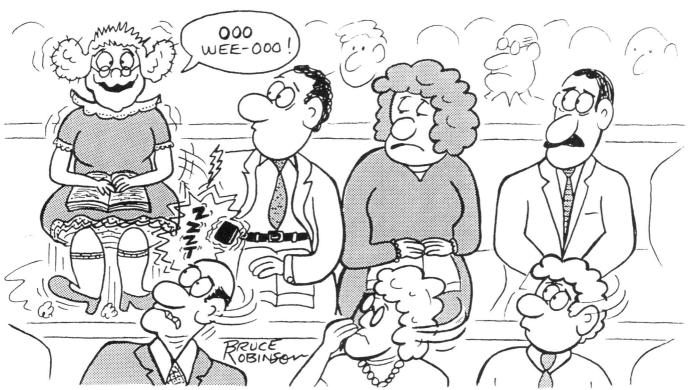

"I told you not to switch your beeper to silent mode."

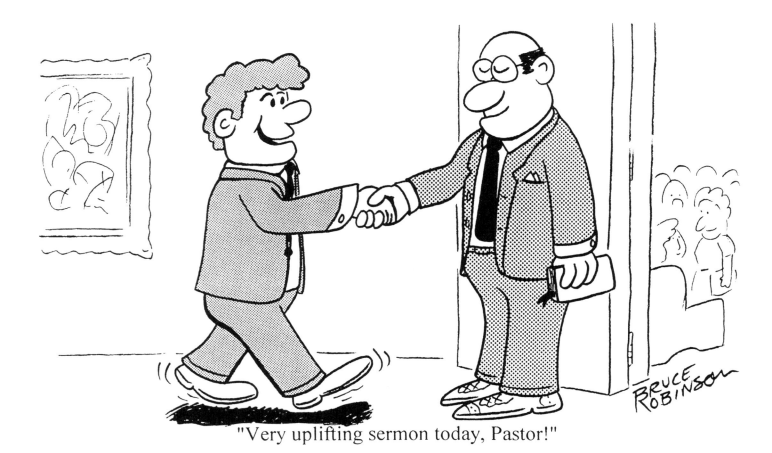

"Very uplifting sermon today, Pastor!"

BRUCE ROBINSON

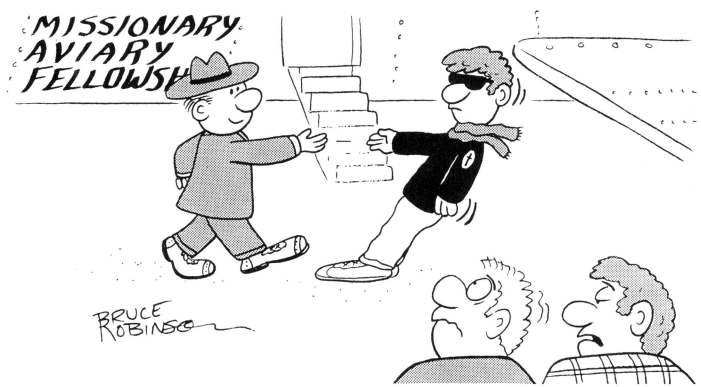

"I hear he just got back from a mission tour of Pisa, Italy."

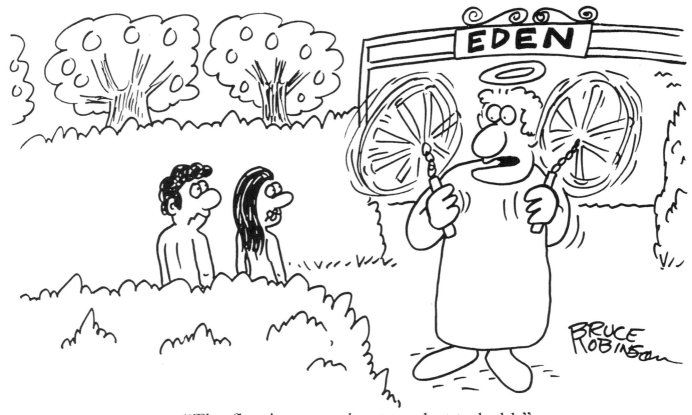

"The flaming sword got too hot to hold."

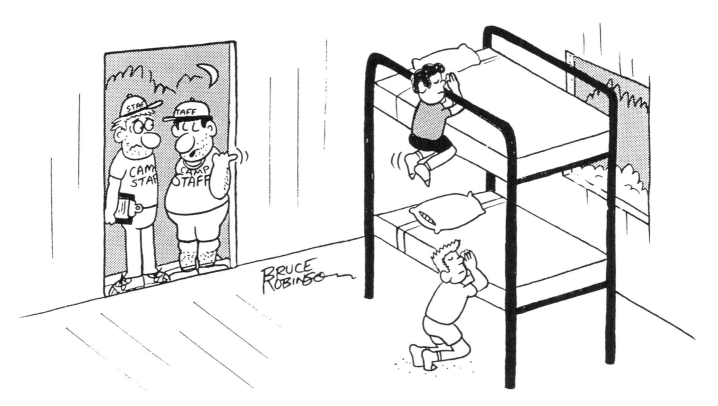

"Now THAT's commitment!"

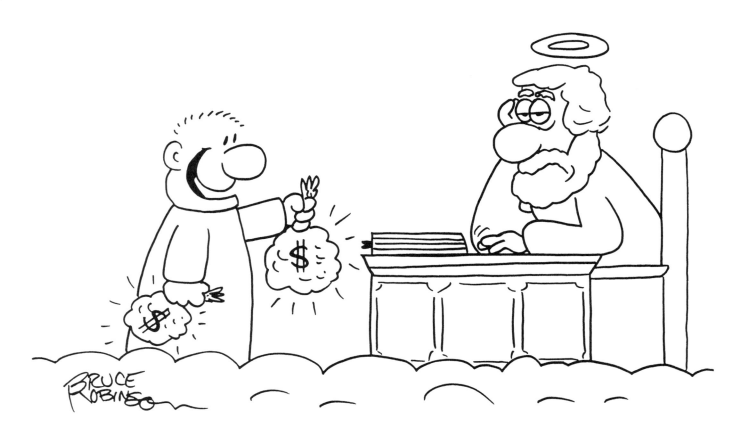

"Are you sure I can't take it with me?...I brought some for **you**..."

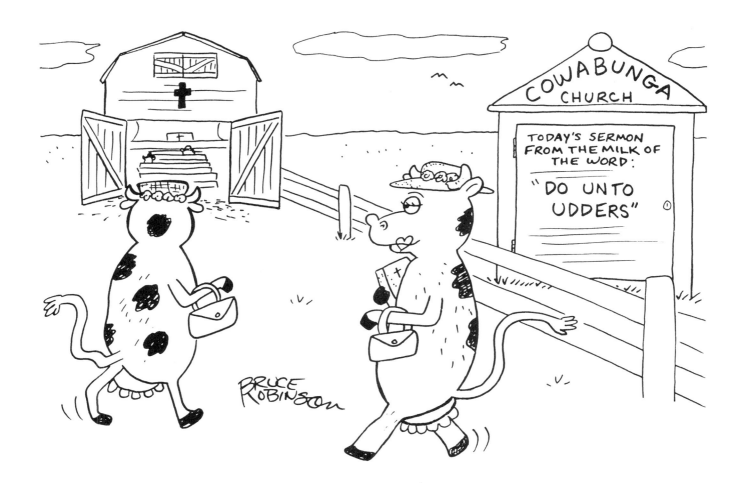

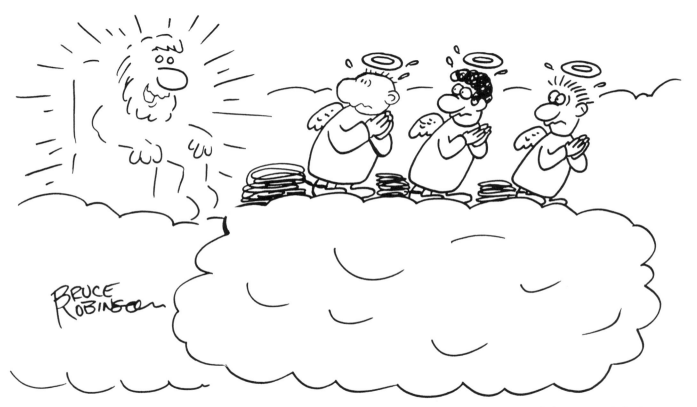

"It's not the Rapture yet, but I want to give the humans something to think about...is everyone ready with their bungee cord?"

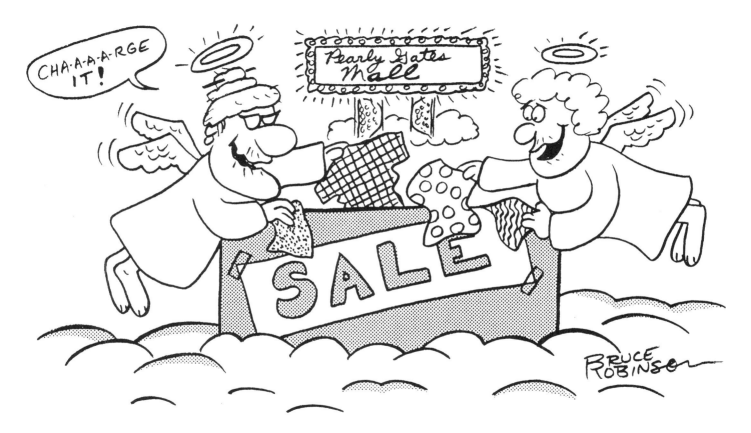

The 'Great Buy and Buy'

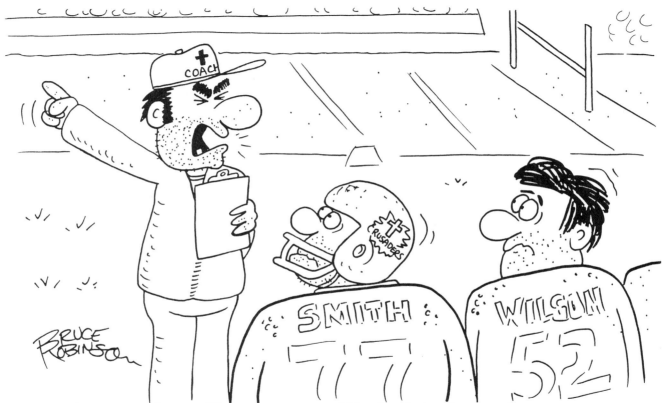

"Remember men-they will know we are His disciples by our love...now get out there and kick some rear-with love."

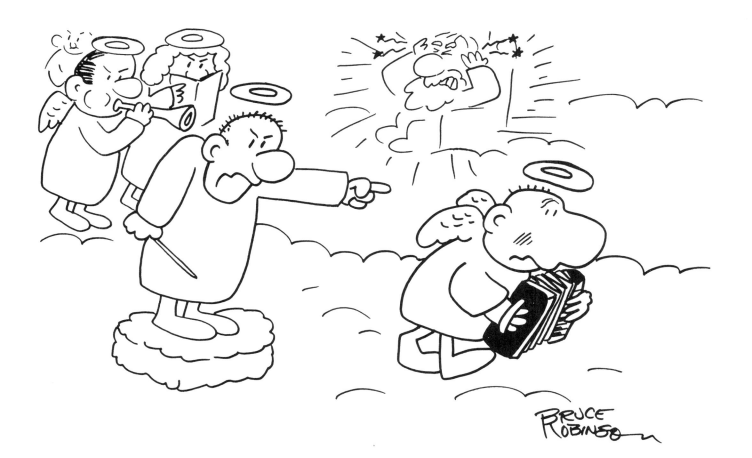

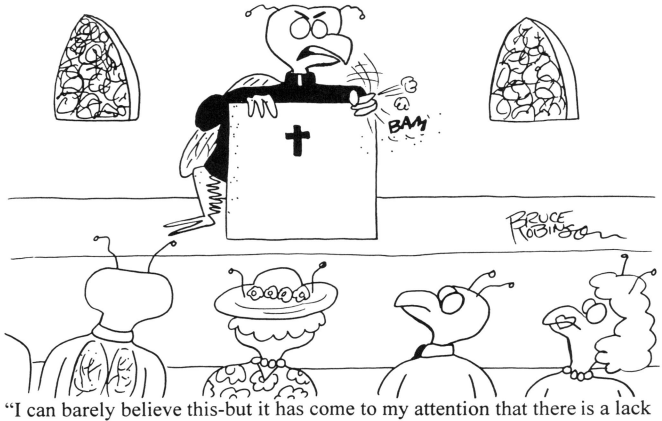

"I can barely believe this-but it has come to my attention that there is a lack of PRAYER in this church!"

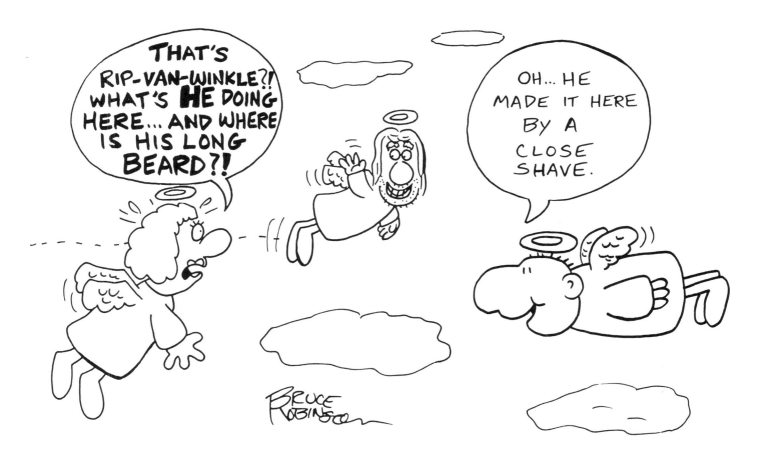

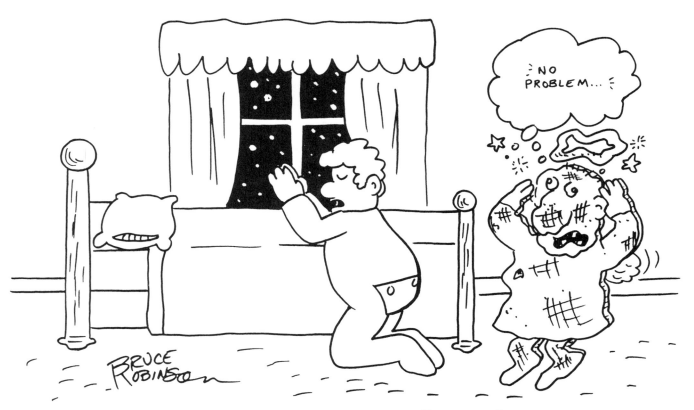

"...and thank you for sending my guardian angel to protect me from that truck today..."

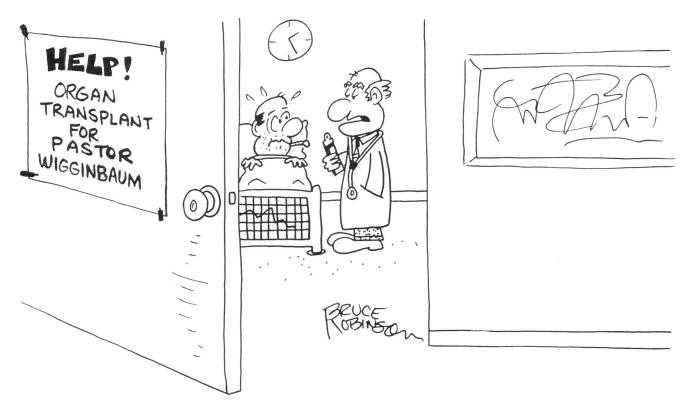

"Bad news, Pastor—the only donation we've gotten so far is a Wurlitzer from the orchestra."

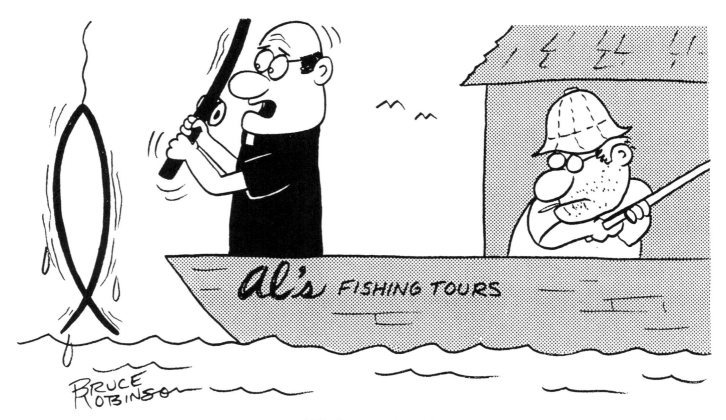

"Holy Mackerel!"

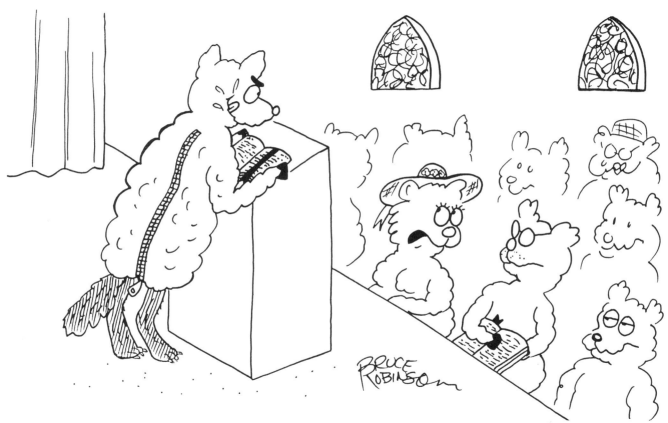

"I don't like the way the new pastor is looking at his flock."

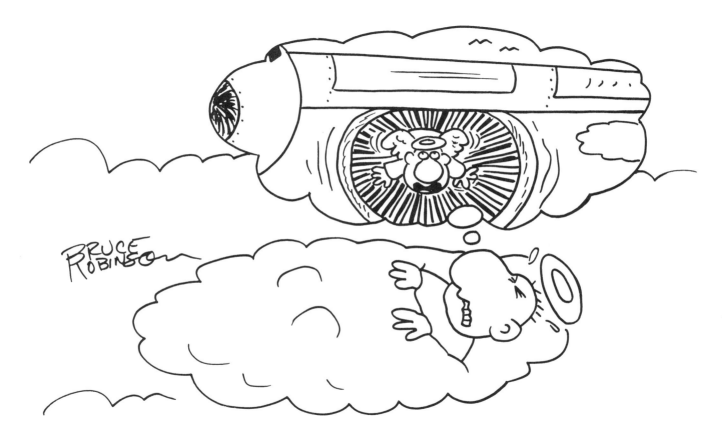

Angel nightmares

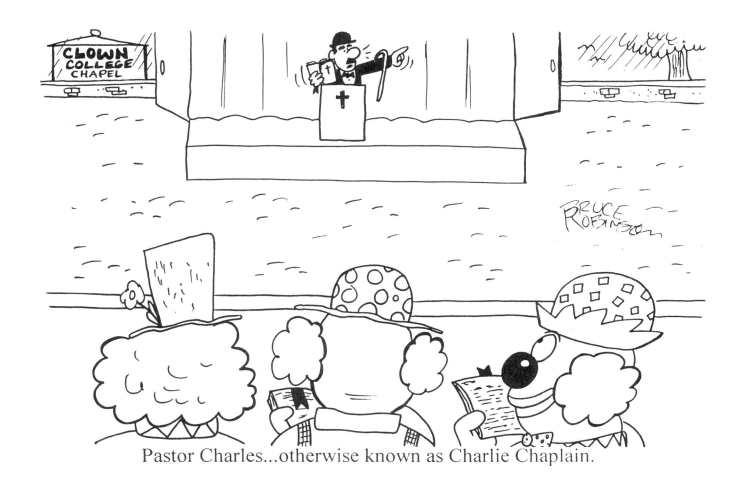

Pastor Charles...otherwise known as Charlie Chaplain.

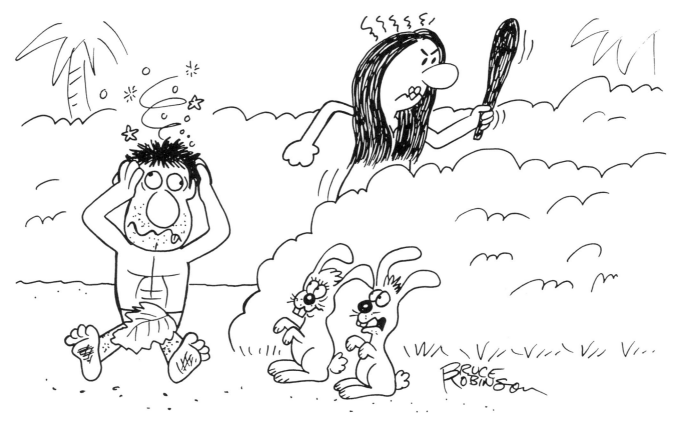

"She just went nuclear and split an Adam!"

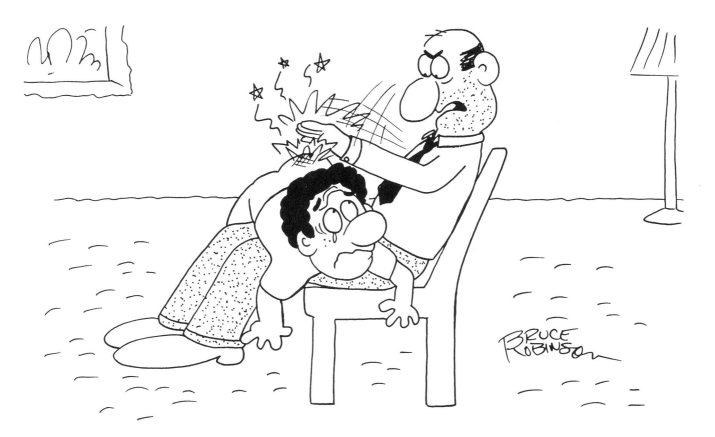

"Now do what the Bible says, and turn the other cheek."

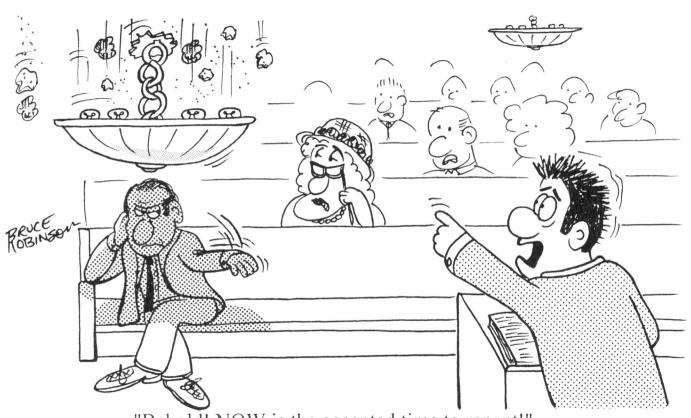

"Behold! NOW is the accepted time to repent!"

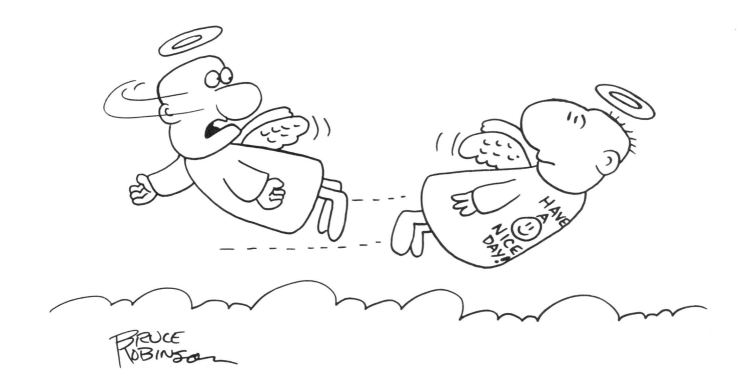

"What other kind of day **is** there up here?!"

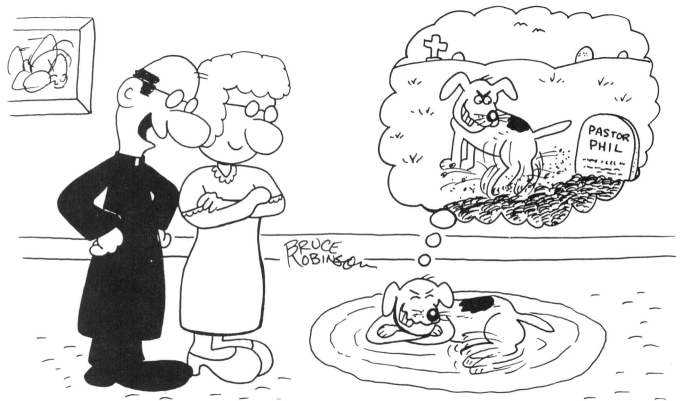

"Heh, heh-good ol' Spot...he must be dreaming about running and playing with me."

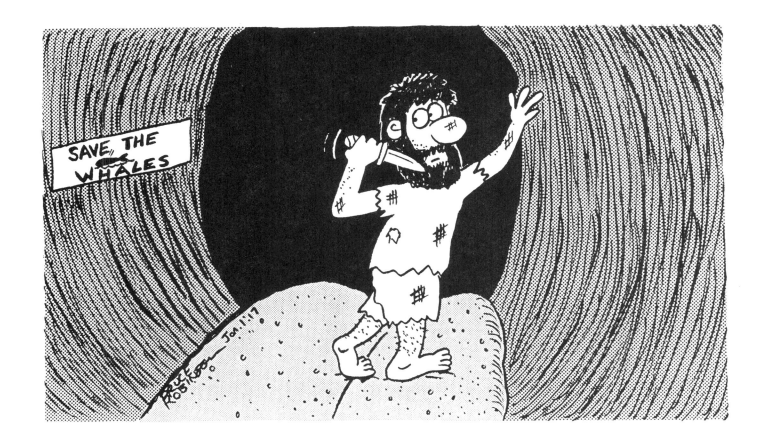

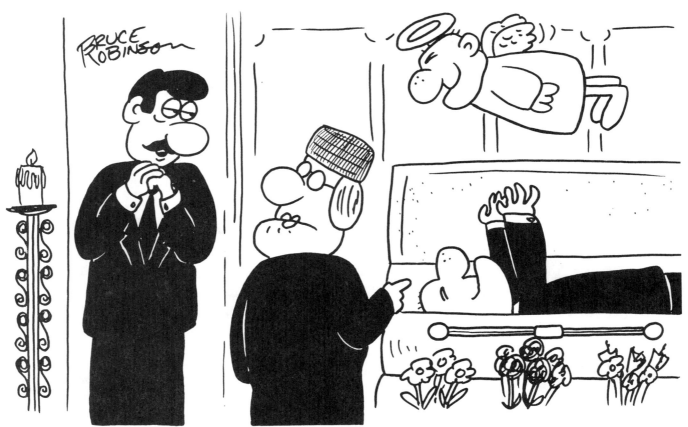

"No...it's not rigormortis...he was Pentacostal."

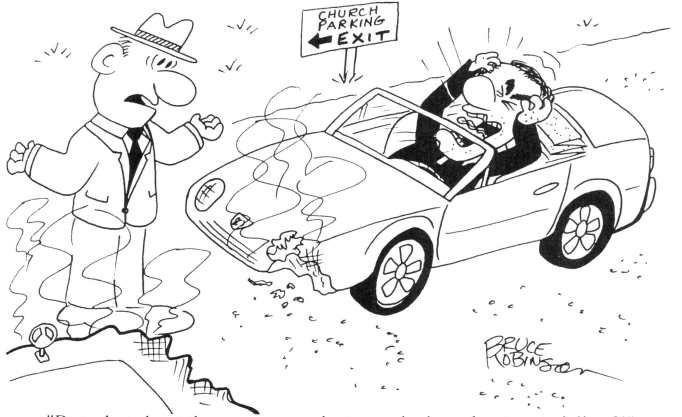

"But what about the sermon you just preached on about materialism?!"

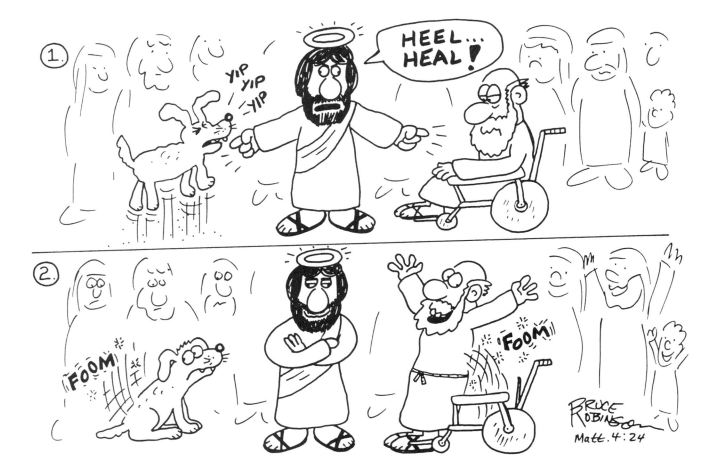

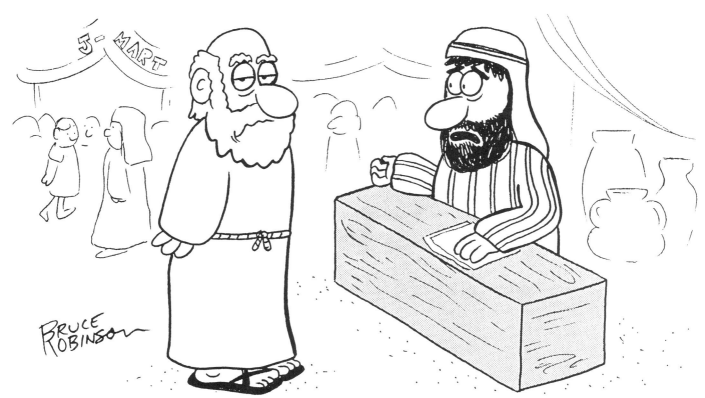

"I'm sorry Noah, we're out of umbrellas-you'll have to take a rain cheque."

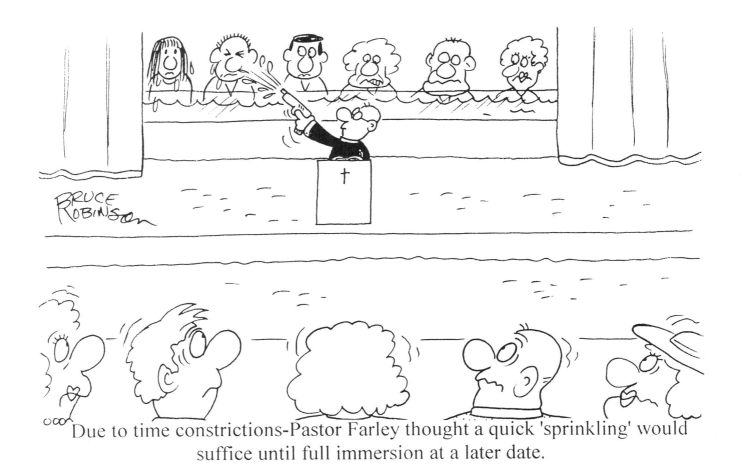

Due to time constrictions-Pastor Farley thought a quick 'sprinkling' would suffice until full immersion at a later date.

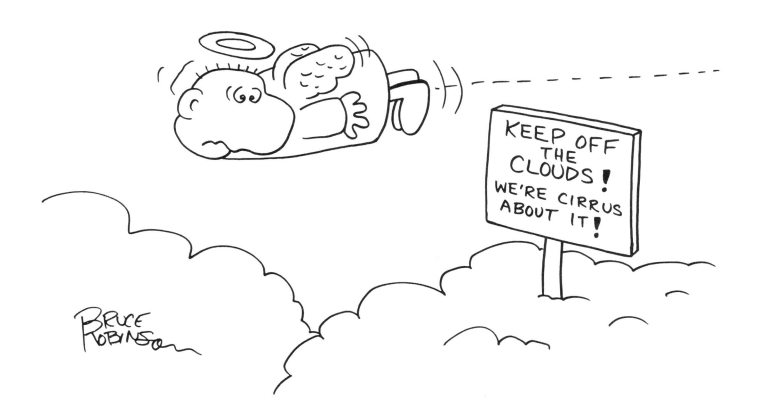

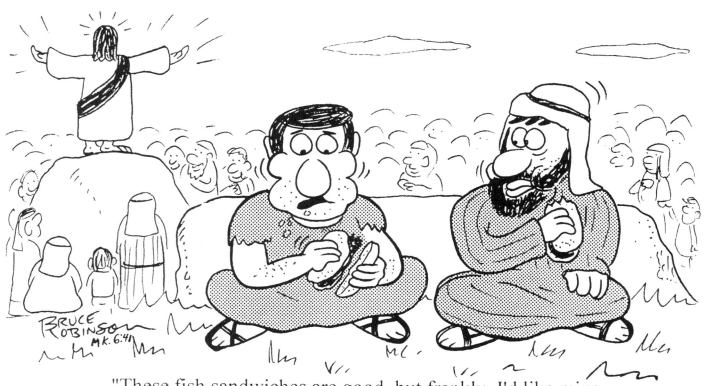

"These fish sandwiches are good, but frankly, I'd like mine with some 'Miracle Whip'."

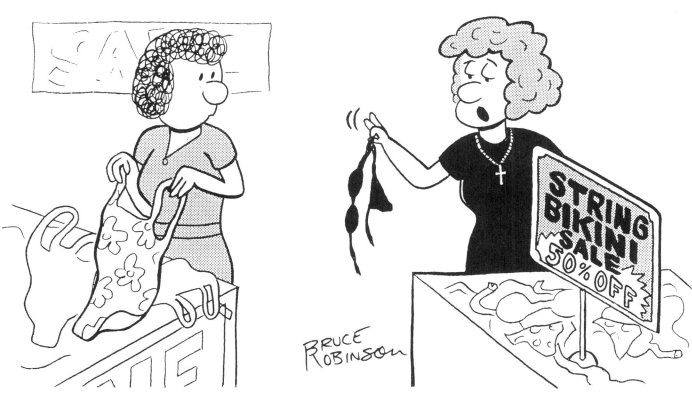

"More like 95% off !"

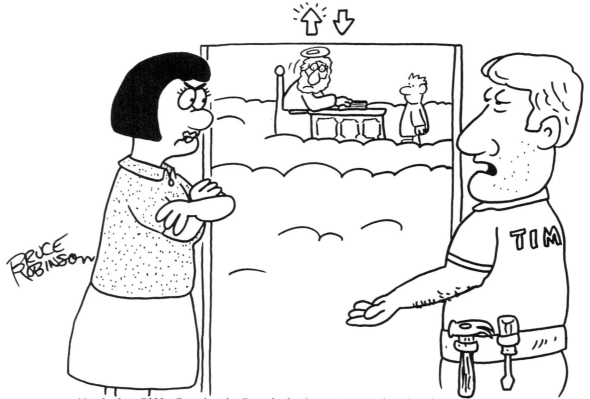

"All right Jill, I admit I might've 'tweaked' the elevator motor a little bit too much."

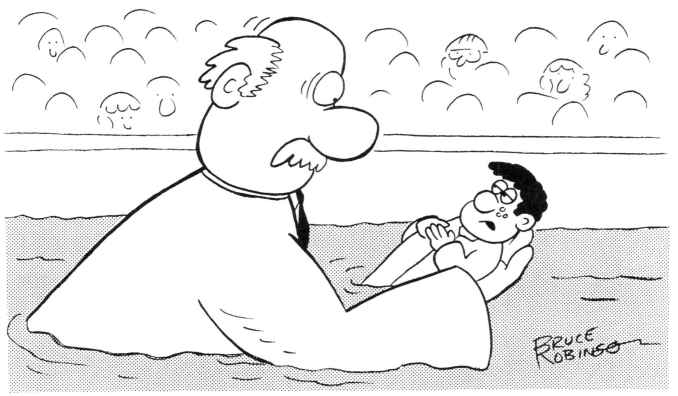

"Yo! You check the 'ph' lately?...I have sensitive eyes, ya know."

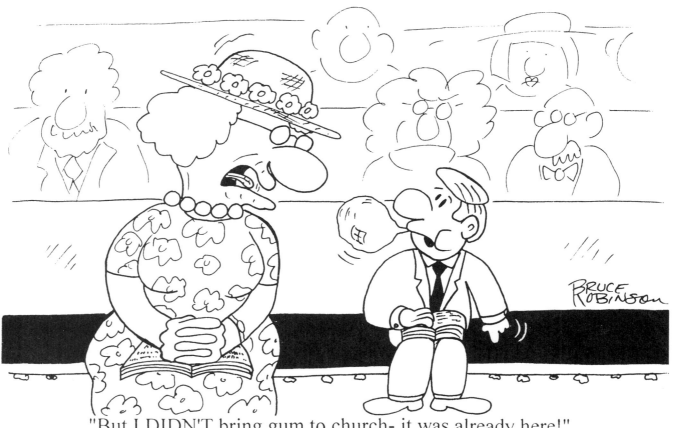

"But I DIDN'T bring gum to church- it was already here!"

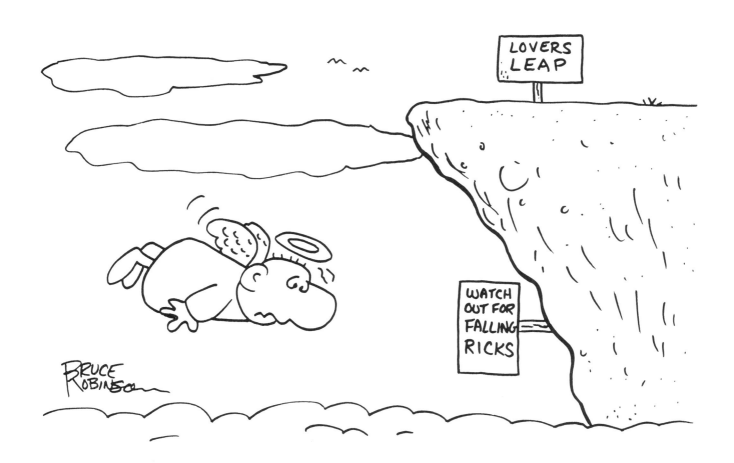

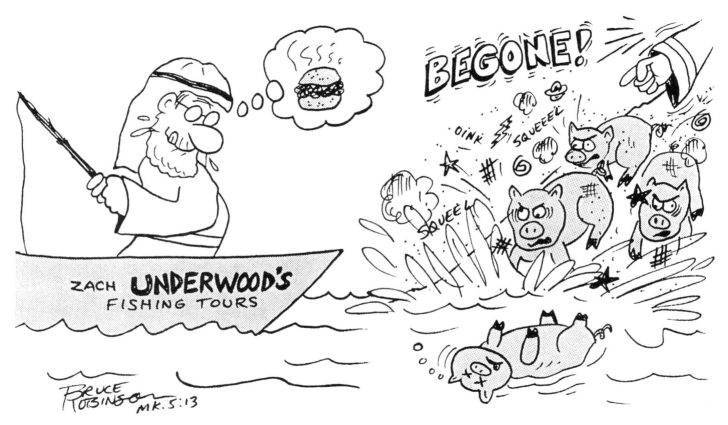

How 'deviled-ham' originated

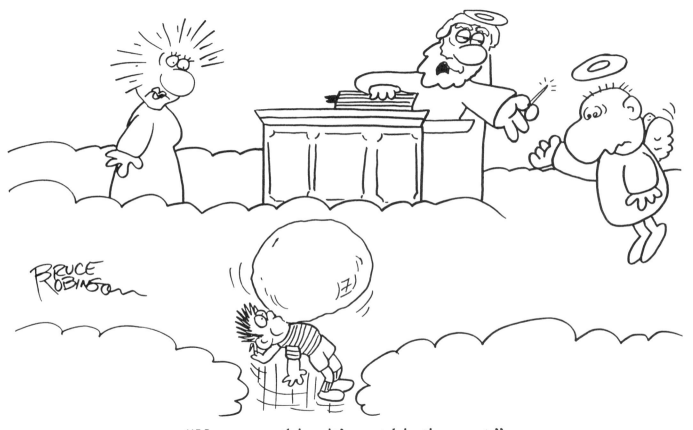

"Here, use this...it's not his time yet."

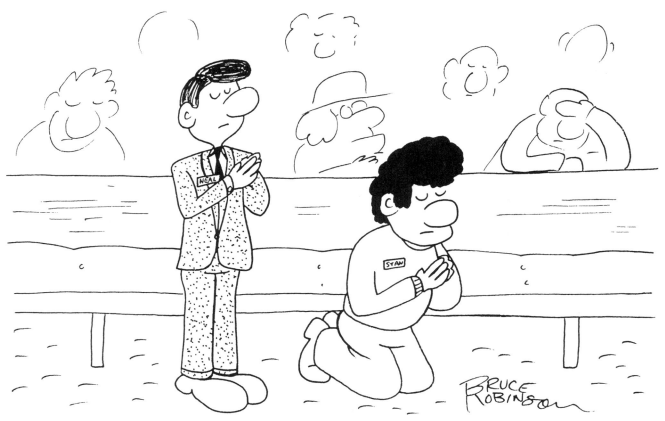

How guys named Neal and Stan, pray.

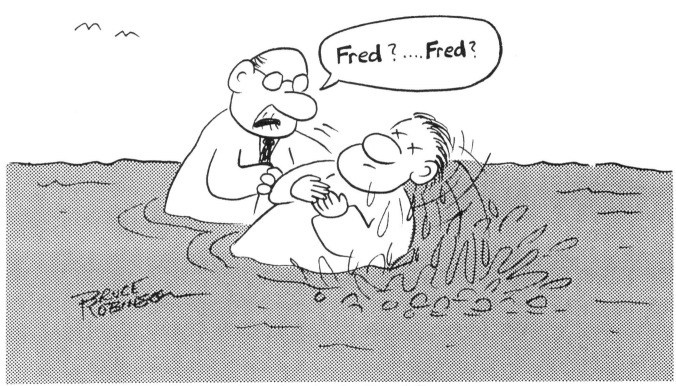

Baptism in the Dead Sea

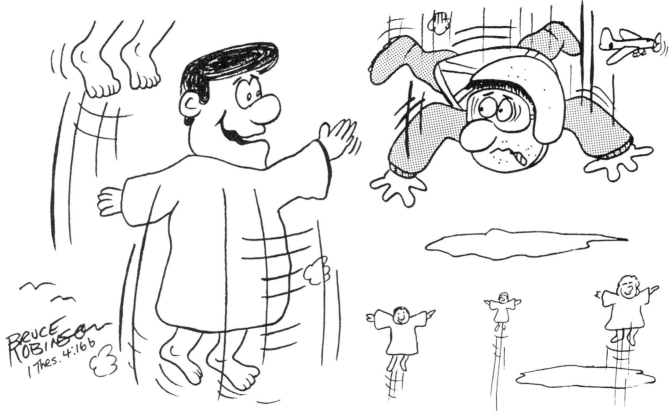

"Reverse Geronimo!"

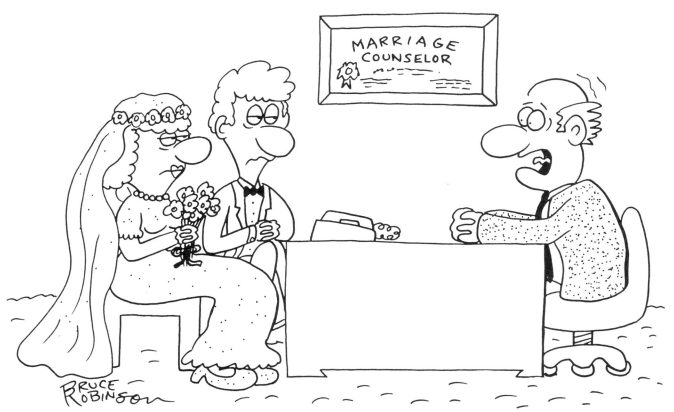

"...and you say the romance has gone out of your marriage?!"

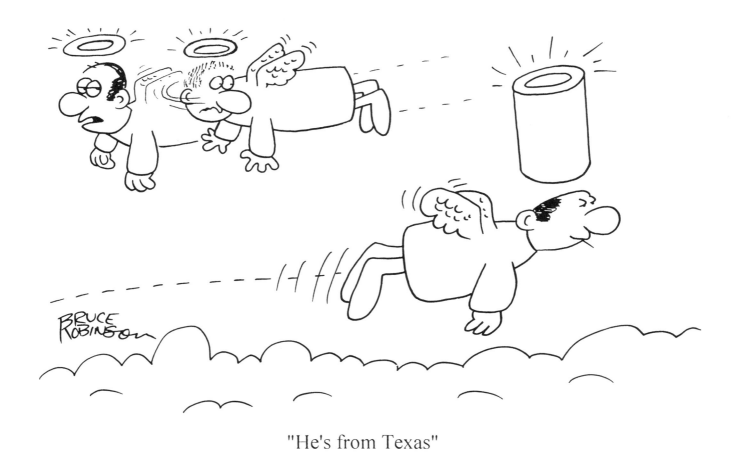

"He's from Texas"

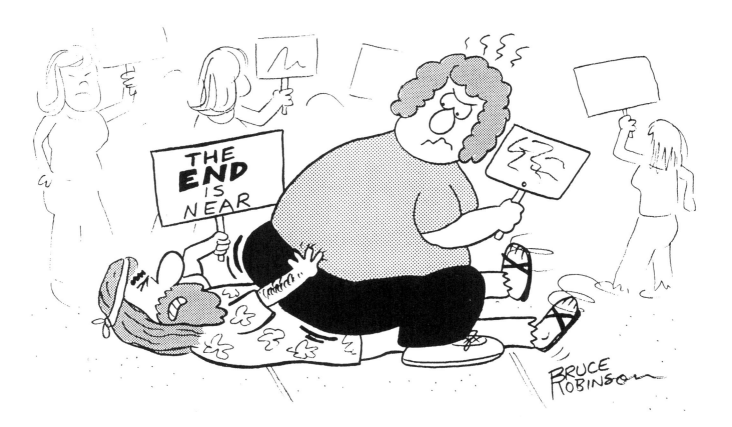

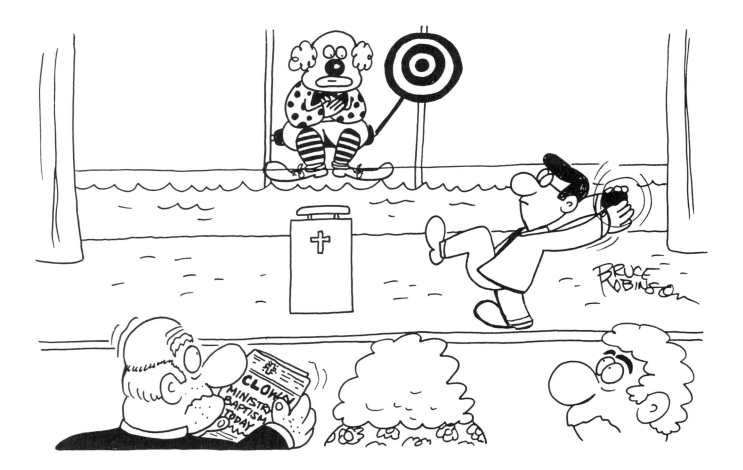

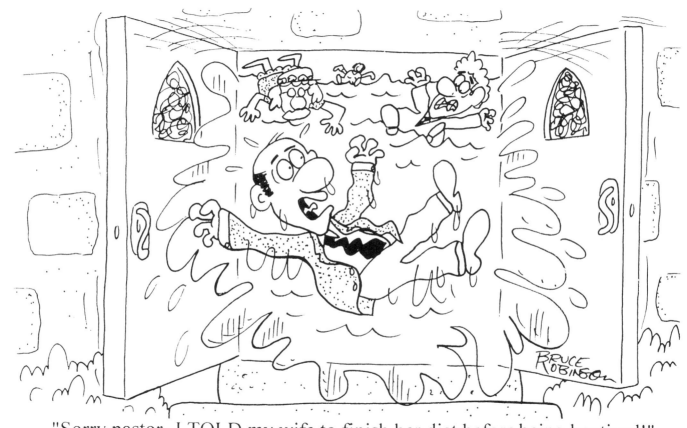

"Sorry pastor- I TOLD my wife to finish her diet before being baptized!"

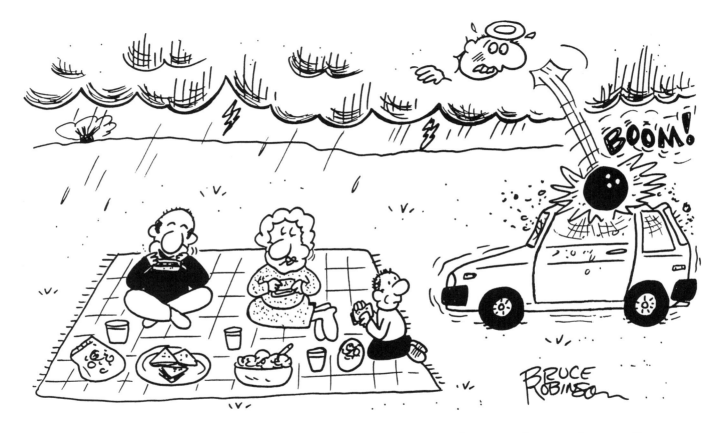

"Heh, heh...'the angels are bowling' is just a figure of speech, son."

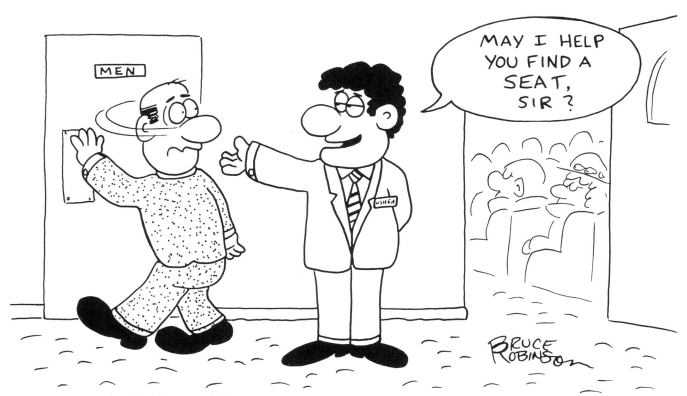

Even though all the positions were filled, Floyd Rabinowitz was convinced his calling was to be an usher- somehow, someway.

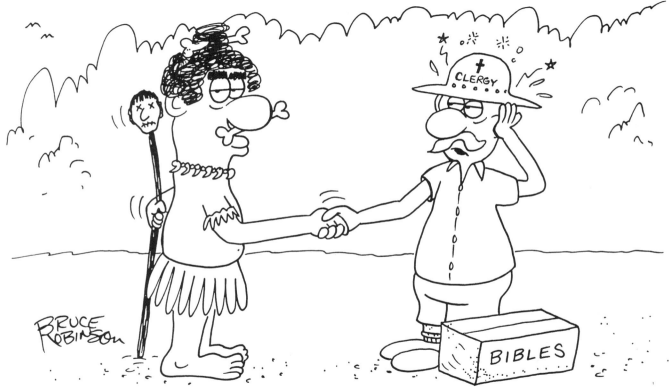

"Nice to meet you chief! By the way ol' chap, do you have anything for a splitting headache?"

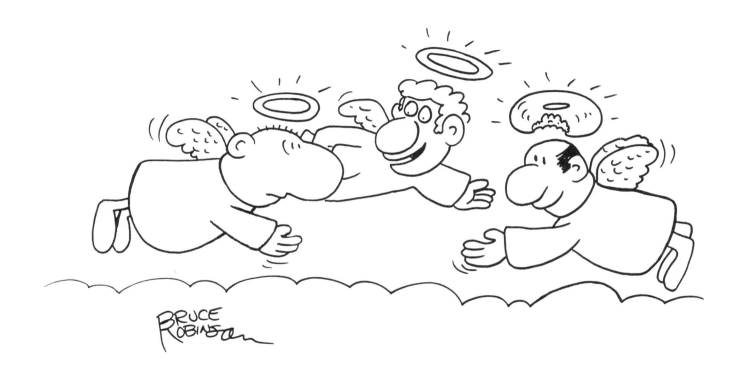

"Harkins, meet Herb...he was in the bagel business."

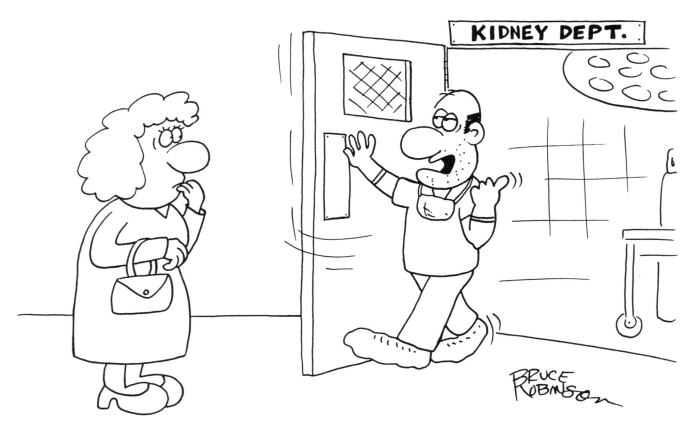

"Pastor Hellfire is recovering well, since he passed his brimstone."

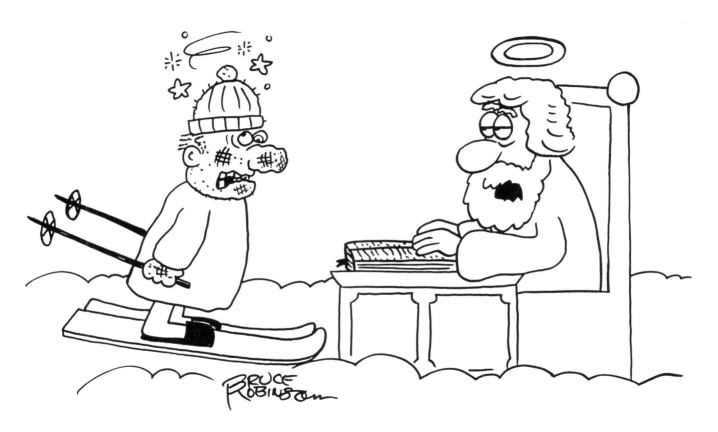

"This is just a temporary visit...you only ran into a rubber tree."

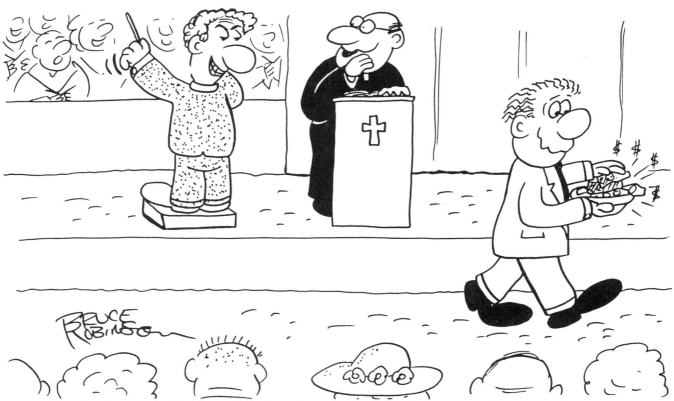

"That, 'I love to tithe' subliminal message on the new offeratory hymn you wrote is really working!"

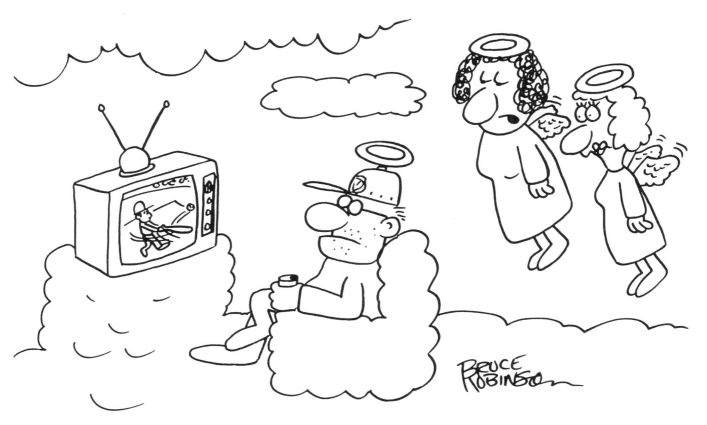

"Since he's been here, he's become a real Padres and Angels fan."

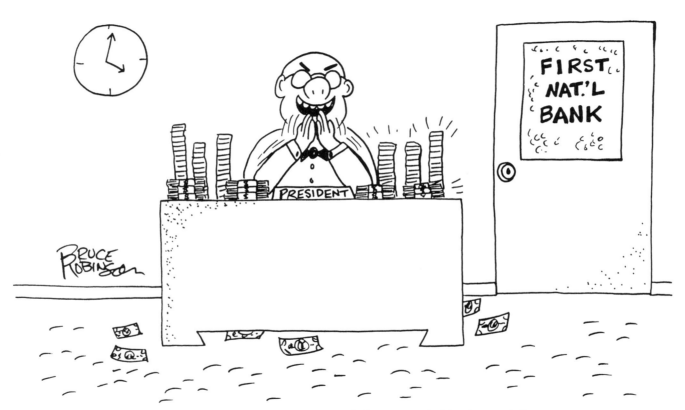

"...and thank you Lord for my daily bread."

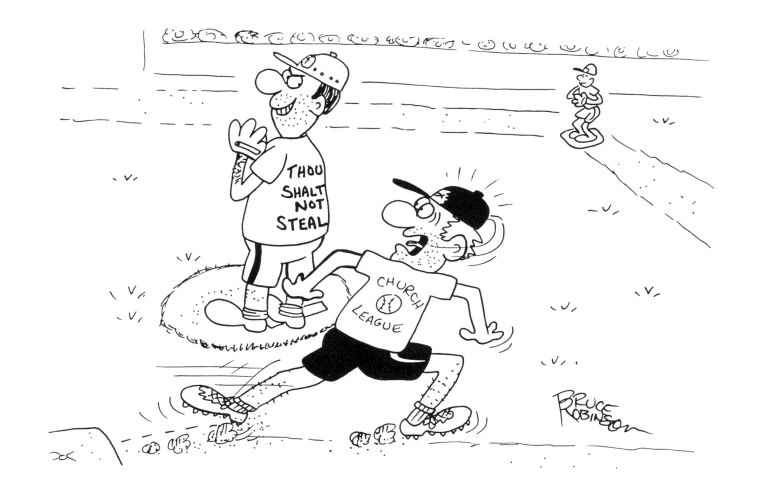

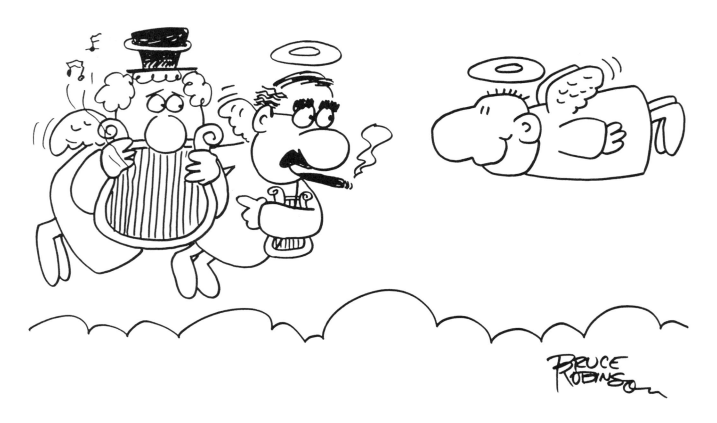

"...and this is my brother, Harpo."

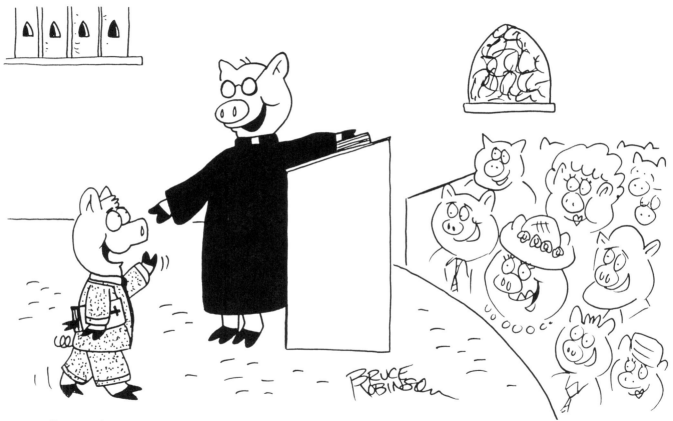

"...and our guest speaker this morning is a missionary to the Pigmies."

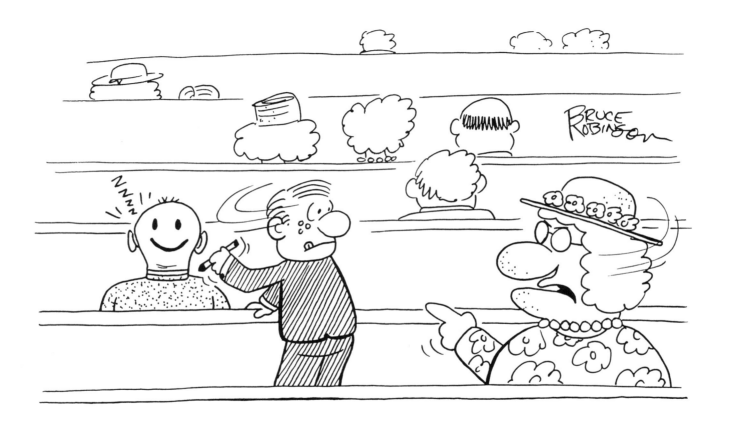

"Billy! Remember grandma said no coloring in church!"

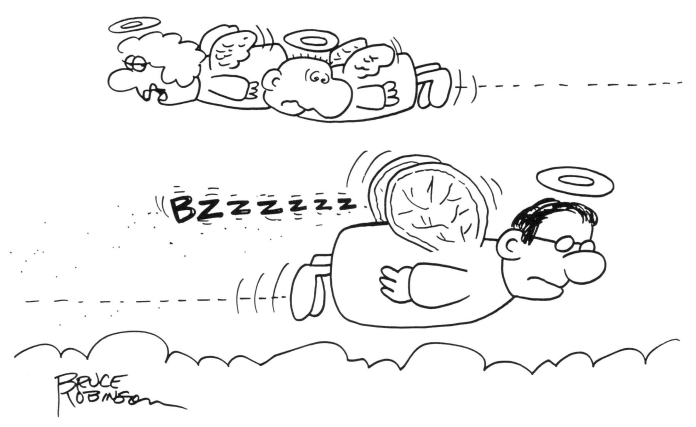

"He used to be an entomologist."

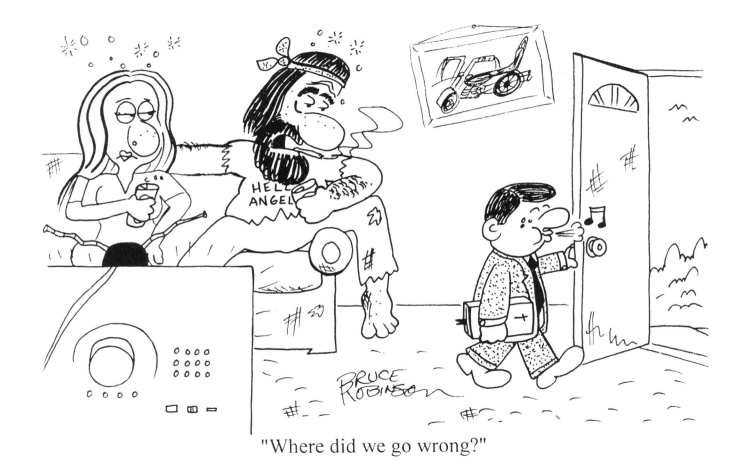

"Where did we go wrong?"

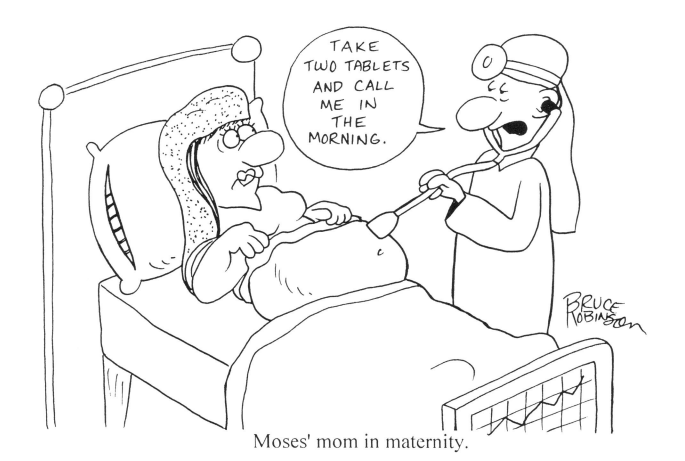

Moses' mom in maternity.

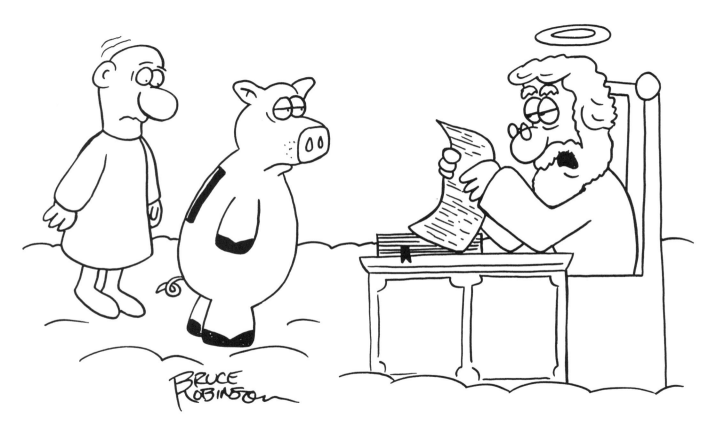

"...says here you were an usher at your church."

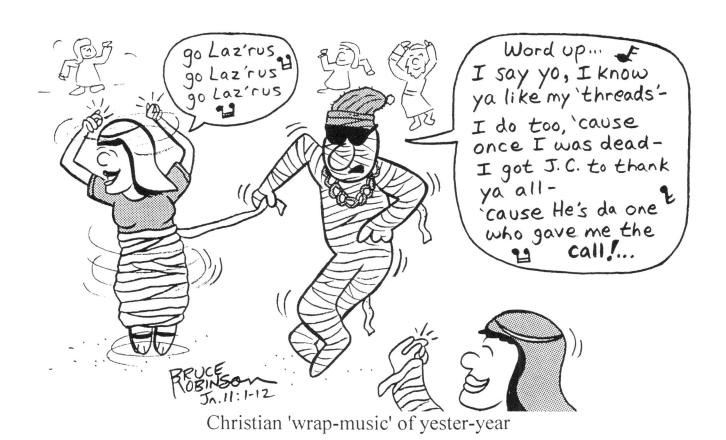

Christian 'wrap-music' of yester-year

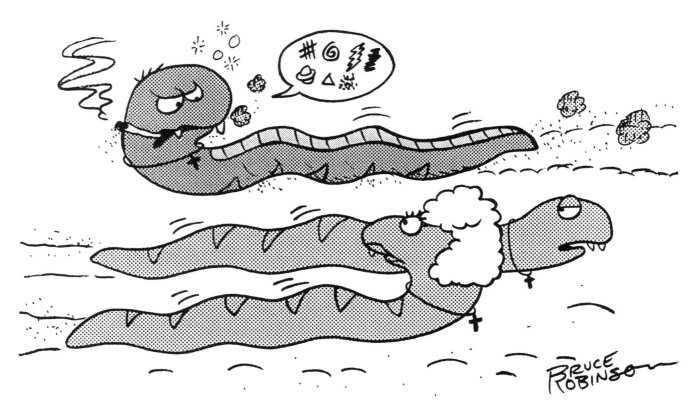

"What a backslider."

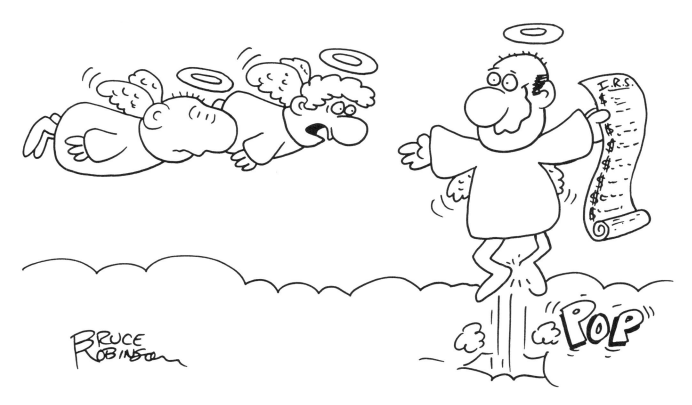

"I heard he had a heart attack while being audited...I guess there really **is** life after debt!"

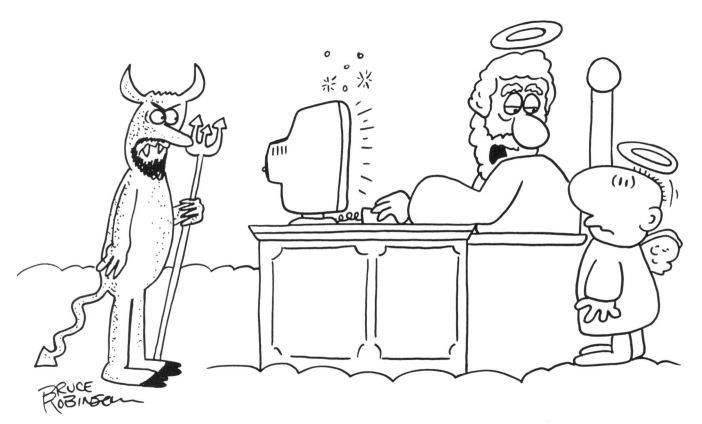

"Tell the Boss we have a **major** computer glitch!"

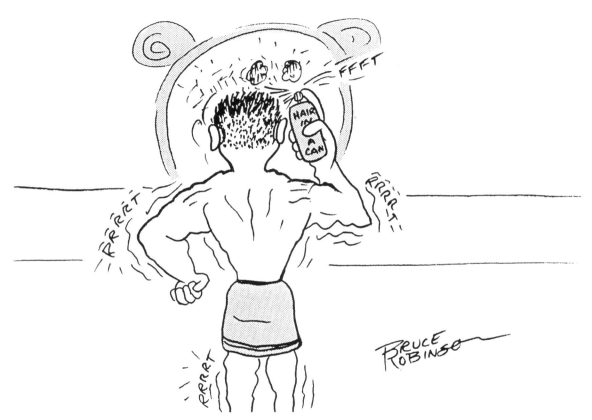

How some say Samson regained his strength

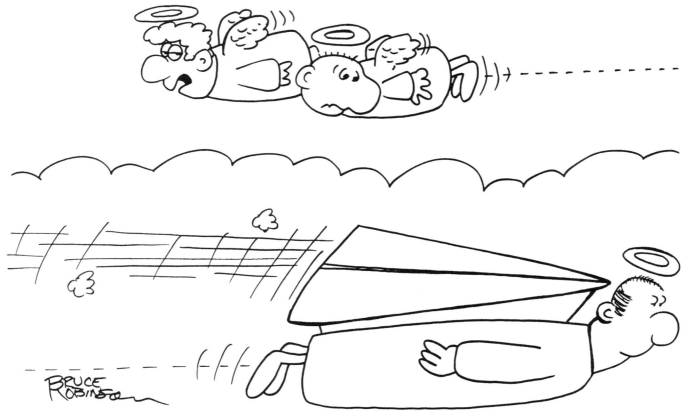

"He used to be an aerodynamics engineer."

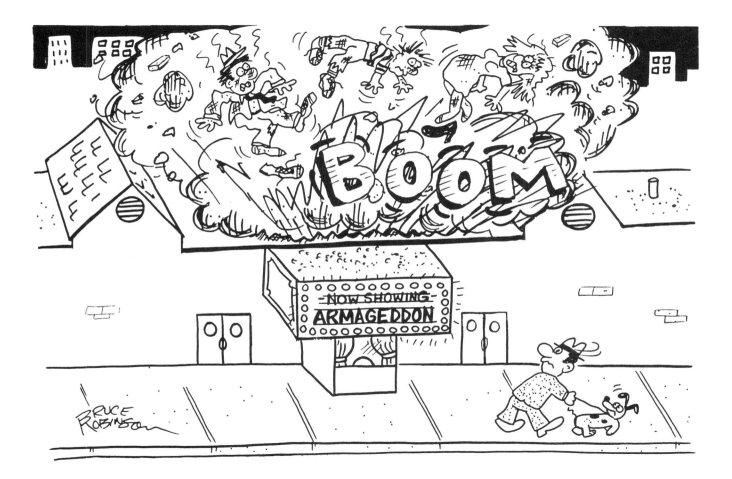

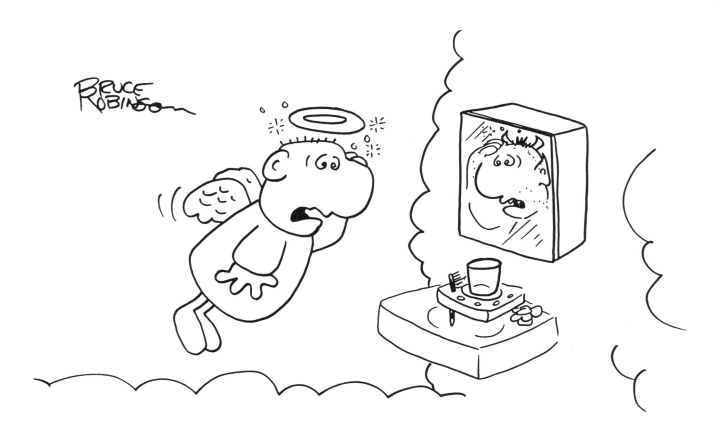

"Man! I gotta cut out those midnight snacks of devils food cake!"

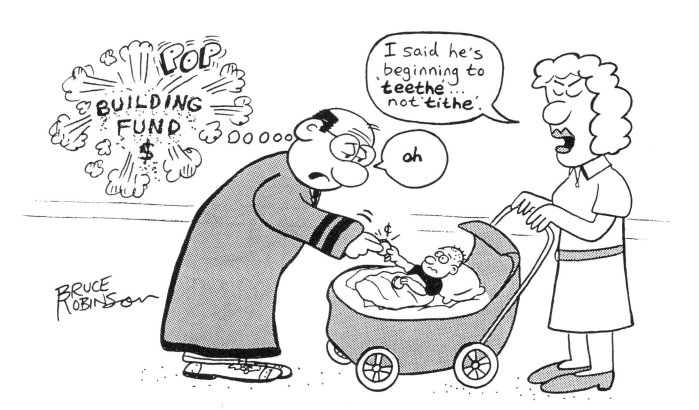

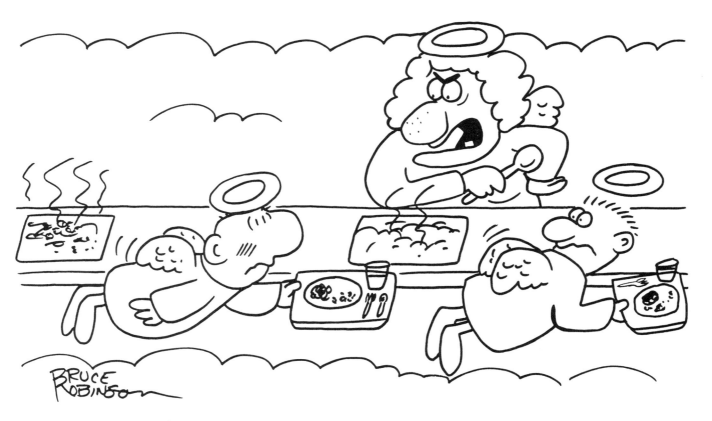

"Deviled eggs, here? What are you, some kinda weirdo?!"

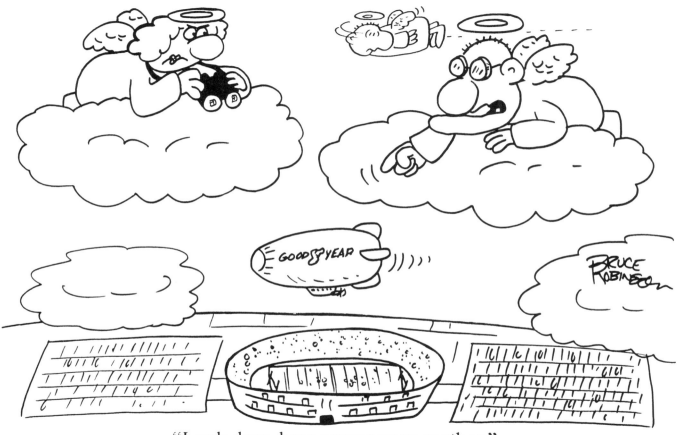

"Look dear, here comes your mother."

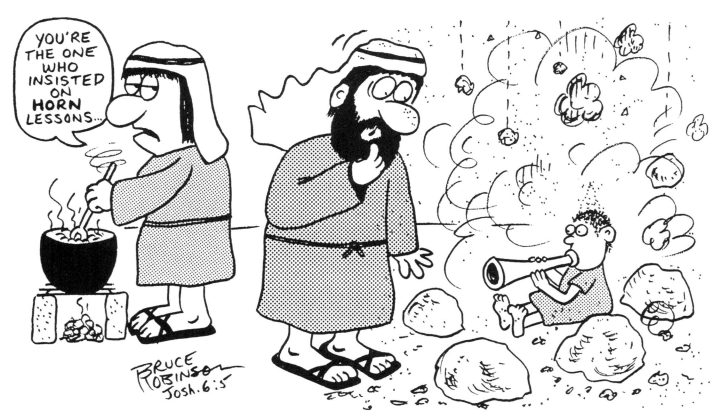

Joshua as a kid

ATTENTION ALL Good Medicine® FANS!

COMING SOON TO A COMPUTER NEAR YOU!

CHECK OUT **Good Medicine**® AT: www.goodmedicine.net

*AND DON'T FORGET TO BECOME AN OFFICIAL MEMBER OF THE Good Medicine®

FAN CLUB !!!

ALL IT TAKES IS A S.A.S.E. (SELF-ADDRESSED STAMPED ENVELOPE) SENT TO: *GOOD MEDICINE c/o BERCO PUBLISHING, INC. 757 S.E. 17 ST. SUITE 399 FT. LAUDERDALE, FL. 33316,* AND YOU'LL GET AN AUTOGRAPHED REPRODUCTION OF THIS BOOK'S FRONT COVER, MADE OUT TO YOU! *PLUS...*YOU'LL GET THE **Good Medicine**® NEWSLETTER, WHICH WILL GIVE YOU THE LATEST SCOOP ON HOW TO GET THE NEWEST & COOLEST **Good Medicine**® MERCHANDISE...INCLUDING *ORIGINAL ART!* SO DON'T DELAY...WRITE TODAY!